Praise for
Yoga Beneath the Surface

"*Yoga Beneath the Surface* is a unique book, and a must read for all serious students. With his extensive knowledge, and profound understanding, Srivatsa Ramaswami makes accessible a broad spectrum of teachings on yoga philosophy and practice. Thinking of Ramaswami, whom I first met in 1974, the words sincerity, humility, and authenticity come to mind. I am grateful to him, and to David Hurwitz, for bringing out this work."

— GARY KRAFTSOW, author of *Yoga for Transformation* and
Yoga for Wellness, founder of American Viniyoga Institute

"David Hurwitz has asked the questions that linger in the mind of many a yoga student but often go unasked. Srivatsa Ramaswami provides insightful answers to a wide variety of issues, including details on the practice of pranayama, advice for dealing with specific issues faced by teachers of yoga, and interesting facts on the philosophy and history of yoga. This book includes something for everyone, and is presented in a narrative, conversational style. David is to be commended for his careful crafting of questions and Srivatsa Ramaswami is to be applauded for his cogent, gentle answers."

— CHRISTOPHER KEY CHAPPLE, professor of
theological studies, Loyola Marymount University

"This book has reached in, grabbed, and tied up so many loose threads for me. David Hurwitz intelligently introduces topics by category and then steps aside to let the master speak clearly to the reader. Conversations on such topics as breath as an uplifting object, breath in asana, meditation on Ishvara, the chikitsa texts, and diagnosis are in depth and sophisticated. Comments on asana practice and karma equally provide implemental treasures for the serious yoga student. The joy of this work is that, in the didactic method of questions and answers that are inherent to the yoga tradition, it offers the serious yoga student user-friendly access to traditional yogic thought. *Yoga Beneath the Surface* has captured the voice, the footprint, and the gentle echoes that will hum in my brain long after my readings."

—VERONICA ZADOR, president of International Association of Yoga Therapists, vice president of Yoga Alliance

"Hollywood writer and life scholar David Hurwitz has turned his attention to yoga. Thank you David! He reveals the vital and sometimes subtle secrets of the great Krishnamacharya, 'the teacher of our teachers.' He shows how you and I as western students can really use yoga to live our lives in peace. David's accord with another great teacher, Srivatsa Ramaswami, in this living lineage of yoga transmission speaks volumes. Ramaswami studied a solid thirty-three years with Krishnamacharya to absorb his gift to the world. David asked his own questions, but has asked them for all of us coming to grips with the questions of What is yoga? and How do I practice in the way that is right for me? Here yoga is made relevant to our present time. Read this book. It reverberates from the ancient source to you."

—MARK WHITWELL, author of *Yoga of Heart*

"A very informative dialogue about yoga off the mat as well as on. Highly recommended for teachers and students of yoga."

—LARRY PAYNE, PhD, coauthor of *Yoga Rx* and *Yoga for Dummies*

"This is a treasure chest full of gems for the serious practitioner and scholar. The book serves as a unique and fascinating guide to the classical tradition that is rarely accessible to the modern student, west or east. The questions by David Hurwitz, a scholar in his own right, are as revealing as the answers by Srivatsa Ramaswami, a modern authority on the traditional written and oral teachings. This is a most humbling, yet equally inspiring book for those of us calling ourselves yoga teachers."

—JOHN KEPNER, director of International Association of Yoga Therapists

YOGA

BENEATH
THE
SURFACE

An American Student and His Indian Teacher
Discuss Yoga Philosophy and Practice

SRIVATSA RAMASWAMI
AND DAVID HURWITZ

MARLOWE & COMPANY
NEW YORK

Yoga Beneath the Surface:
An American Student and His Indian Teacher Discuss Yoga Philosophy and Practice

Copyright © 2006 by Srivatsa Ramaswami and David Hurwitz
Photographs copyright © 2004 by Srivatsa Ramaswami

Published by
Marlowe & Company
An Imprint of Avalon Publishing Group, Incorporated

AVALON

Library of Congress Cataloging-in-Publication Data
Ramaswami, Srivatsa.
Yoga beneath the surface : an American student and his Indian teacher discuss
yoga philosophy and practice / Srivatsa Ramaswami and David Hurwitz.
p. cm.
Includes bibliographical references and index.
ISBN 1-56924-294-1 (pbk.)
1. Hatha yoga. 2. Yoga—Philosophy. 3. Yoga—Miscellanea.
I. Hurwitz, David. II. Title.
RA781.7.R33 2006
613.7'046—dc22
2006007830

ISBN-13: 978-1-56924-294-0

9 8 7 6 5 4 3 2 1

Designed by Pauline Neuwirth, Neuwirth & Associates, Inc.

Printed in the United States of America

To the fond memories of my generous guru,
Sri. T. Krishnamacharya
—SRIVATSA RAMASWAMI

To my wife, Jane, who stuck with me through it all.
—DAVID HURWITZ

Disclaimer

ALL YOGA SHOULD be practiced under the guidance of a qualified teacher. All medical conditions should be treated by a qualified doctor. Nothing in this book is meant to be prescriptive for any ailment or condition. Nothing in this book is meant to replace either a yoga teacher or a medical doctor.

Please note that not all exercises mentioned in this book are suitable for everyone, and any exercise program may result in injury. Please be sure to consult your physician before beginning any exercise program. While the authors and the publisher have tried to ensure that the exercises discussed in this book are accurate and safe, they are not responsible for adverse effects or consequences sustained by anyone using the book. No liability shall attach to the authors or publisher for loss or damage of any nature suffered as a result of reliance on the reproduction of any of this book's contents or any errors or omissions herein.

Contents

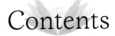

X

Acknowledgments

MY SINCERE THANKS to my wife, Uma, for her continued support, to my son, Badri, and his wife, Audrey, for their support and hosting us during all these extended visits; my son Prasanna and his wife Tina for their continued support and encouragement. Many thanks to Matthew Lore, the publisher, and Peter Jacoby, of Marlowe & Company, for publishing and editing this book. To Bob Silverstein, for acting as the literary agent for this publication, my sincere thanks are due. Thanks are also due to my young friends, Tatyana Papova, Girija, Klaus Koenig, Ranjit Babu, Dr. Mahendran, Kirti, and Tiruchelvan, for giving their yoga pictures for use in the book.

—SRIVATSA RAMASWAMI

∾&

MY INDEBTEDNESS AND gratitude to Ramaswami are without measure. I thank him for his beautiful answers and for his patience with my questions.

For help in shaping my early ideas on the subject I thank my previous teachers in this lineage: Gary Kraftsow, A. G. Mohan, and Larry Payne. Also Desikachar and Kausthub, for the many workshops of theirs I attended.

To my fellow Ramaswami students, Vivian Richman and Tonya

Riley, for letting me use some of their own questions along with his answers.

To my wife, Jane Sindell, and my colleagues Pam Hoxsey, Vivian, and Mark Whitwell for their support all through the project, especially for reading early drafts and sharing their comments.

To Matthew Lore of Marlowe & Company, for publishing the book.

To our editor, Peter Jacoby, for his thoughtful notes and ideas for making the book more accessible.

To our agent, Bob Silverstein, of Quicksilver Books, for his help and advice.

—DAVID HURWITZ

Preface

I HAD SPENT considerable time contemplating my earlier books before deciding to start writing them. But, with this book, I did not even realize that I was in the process of writing a book until after it was almost half written: When David Hurwitz (known as "Yogi Dave" among his yoga colleagues) started sending me questions in fits and starts, and asked me if I would care to answer some of them, I agreed, basically because his questions were very thought provoking and sincere. I also found him to be one of the rare yogis of modern times who have an abiding interest and competence not only in the physical aspects of yoga but also in its spiritual and philosophical dimensions. Our dialogue eventually produced sufficient material to be published as this book.

I met Yogi Dave for the first time when I was teaching Bhakti yoga at a seminar. I marveled at the way that he asked very pertinent questions about Bhakti or Vinyasa yoga. Then we met on several other occasions, at John Coon's Yoga Center in Houston, at Yoga Works in L.A., and subsequently at Loyola Marymount University. Over a two-year period, we discussed several aspects of yoga: details of vinyasa krama (movement and sequence), different sutras (concise statements), the chikitsa (therapeutic) approach to yoga. He had a very good understanding of my guru Sri. T. Krishnamacharya's approach to yoga, as he had also studied with some of Krishnamacharya's senior students, and studied their works as well. It has been a great pleasure working with David Hurwitz.

The topics covered here are wide ranging. I hope yoga students who may have similar questions will find this work useful.

—SRIVATSA RAMASWAMI

✑

WHAT A SURPRISE and delight it was for me to meet Srivatsa Ramaswami.

Since 1990, I have been studying the yoga tradition of T. Krishnamacharya (now passed on), the great south Indian yogi who lived in Madras (now Chennai). I was lucky enough to study with one of Krishnamacharya's senior Indian students and with the American disciple of another, both here in the United States and in Madras, over a period of ten years. This tradition flowing from Krishnamacharya was the tradition I connected with most, and about which I wanted to learn more. It is yoga as it was classically taught, without the many so-called innovations we find today under the rubric of "creativity."

Then, one day in 2000, I was surfing the Net. I must have typed in the keywords "Krishnamacharya" and "yoga." And the name that popped up was Srivatsa Ramaswami. He had been teaching in Chicago, and I read a review of his workshop. I could hardly believe it. This man, whom I had never heard of, had studied with Krishnamacharya for over three decades. Of course I wanted to meet him.

In November 2000, Srivatsa Ramaswami revisited the United States, for a yoga conference in Austin, Texas, where he taught a workshop in *bhakti* (devotion). It was there that I met him for the first time. When he explained the three different times *ishvara pranidhana* (surrender to God) occurs in the *Yoga Sutras of Patan-jali* (the classic yoga text), I was enthralled. I could immediately see the breath and scope of his knowledge. I introduced myself and asked a few questions. I have been asking him questions on yoga ever since—and, he has been answering them!

That Ramaswami had studied for over thirty years with Krish-namacharya became clear very quickly. The tradition runs deep in him, and pours out effortlessly. His mastery of the yoga texts and scriptures is impressive. His chanting is quite beautiful and engaging. The way he teaches asana is related, but different, from what I had learned before.

The asana method he uses is called vinyasa krama—sequence and movement—and this was the way Krishnamacharya had taught asanas (yogic poses). I learned that the vinyasa krama method is quite logical: Each asana is in a sequence leading to the next. Each asana helps your body, mind, and breathing to learn the main asana of the sequence. I also learned that the method is com-prehensive: There are over seven hundred vinyasas (variations) of asanas, many of which I cannot do. But, as Ramaswami would point out, it is important to be able to teach students who are more flexible than one is. So he teaches the full range of asanas—always emphasizing how much of yoga goes beyond asana, how the real goal of yoga is to know the true nature of the self.[1]

After meeting Ramaswami in Austin, I bought and studied his first book, *Yoga for the Three Stages of Life*. It is the most complete portrait that I have come across of what it means to be a yogi in south India. And we stayed in touch. In 2001, when I was again in Madras, I visited him in his home, met his wife, Uma, and chatted for an afternoon. I hoped someday he would become my teacher.

---

[1] This is the goal of yoga according to the sage Patanjali, whose text Krishnamacharya took to be the ultimate authority on the subject. It differs from the goal of Hatha yoga, which is to unite the two energies symbolically represented by the sun (ha) and the moon (tha). Do these two goals amount to the same thing? A good ques-tion indeed.

Eventually, he did. I traveled to Houston, when he was there; we had group classes and many private sessions together. I arranged for him to come to Los Angeles, where I live, for more classes and private sessions. He was patient and generous, holding nothing back. I learned a great deal from him and it changed my practice. My asana practice is now vinyasa krama. My basis for studying continues to be the *Yoga Sutras of Patanjali*.

After his second trip to Los Angeles, where he taught a month-long course in vinyasa krama at Loyola University, Ramaswami's second book, *The Complete Book of Vinyasa Yoga*, came out. It gives a detailed exposition of the vinyasa krama methodology.

As I continued to practice and study yoga, I encountered more and more techniques and ideas. I came to feel my situation was not unique. Other yoga students must be traversing similar terrain, especially other American students trying to understand a philosophy and methodology coming from a foreign country and passed down from long ago.

And so, in July 2003, knowing that many classic Indian texts (such as the *Yoga Yajnavalkya*, a dialogue between husband and wife) were written in question-and-answer format, I suggested we create a book of our own questions and answers about yoga. Ramaswami liked the idea and we set to work. I had already asked many questions, and I had many more to ask. During that year and the next, I submitted batch after batch of questions to Ramaswami, and he promptly returned his quite beautiful answers. The innovation of e-mail proved remarkably helpful to us. This book is the result.

Ramaswami's answers were written in his "Indian English," in a conversational tone, much as he would have answered them in a class. I have corrected these for clarity, and added some punctuation where needed. But my desire has been to preserve the original "authentic" flavor of the answers, so I have not tried to overcorrect them or turn them into proper-sounding American English.

I think the content should prove stimulating and illuminating to the many students of yoga who have tried, on their own, to dive beneath the surface of some of the many facets of this ancient practice. Enjoy, and remember to exhale.

—DAVID HURWITZ

Introduction

HOW DO WE achieve the famous *ahimsa* (nonviolence)? Is it an act of will or something we can practice? How does the yogi "see" his *purusha* (soul)? Does the yogi die in *samadhi* (absorption)? What role does walking play in yoga? What should you do about your yoga practice when traveling? What is the role of breath in asana? Of *bandha* (lock) in asana? Where does willpower come in? Was Krishnamacharya happy? What if a student only has half an hour to practice?

This book contains almost 250 questions on the various aspects of yoga, each of which is followed by Ramaswami's answer. Most of the questions come from our practice and study together, along with questions arising from reading the reference texts listed on page 247. A few came from colleagues and students. The questions were originally asked in random order. Later, we organized them according to subject. This, of course, can only be an approximation, for many of the answers touch on several topics and fall under several headings. The untidiness of real conversation frequently pierces the attempt at logical organization.

The texts we refer to were chosen, in the first place, from among those Ramaswami studied with Krishnamacharya, the two classics: the *Yoga Sutras of Patanjali* and the *Hatha Yoga Pradipika* (Light on Hatha Yoga), and two somewhat lesser-known texts that were nevertheless very important to Krishnamacharya: *The Yoga Rahasya* [Secret of Yoga] *of Nathamuni* (a ninth-century yogi) and *The Yoga*

Yajnavalkya (Yajnavalkya was a sage). And, of course, as teacher and student, we turned frequently to the two books written by Ramaswami himself: *Yoga for the Three Stages of Life* and *The Complete Book of Vinyasa Yoga*.

✺ CONTENTS AND STRUCTURE ✺ OF THIS BOOK

The Ashtanga (eight-limbs) yoga of Patanjali is the subject of most of the questions and answers in this book. So it seemed natural for the chapters of this book to roughly correspond to the eight limbs, namely:

- *yamas* (don'ts)
- *niyama* (dos)
- *asana* (posture)
- *pranayama* (yogic breath control)
- *pratyahara* (starving the senses)
- *dharana* (concentration)
- *dhyana* (meditation
- *samadhi* (absorption)

Because *swadhyaya* (study of the scriptures), is included as one of the niyamas, we have placed the topic of yoga philosophy first. Next come the chapters on asana, pranayama, and meditation. (Because dharana, dhyana, and samadhi are different degrees of the process usually labeled meditation, we have included those discussions in the meditation chapter.)

We conclude the book with two additional topics, a chapter on yoga therapy and another on everyday matters (which includes some of Ramaswami's personal reflections on his teacher, Krishnamacharya).

At the core of yoga philosophy is the answer to the questions: Who am I? What is the true nature of the self (*purusha*)? How do you come to know your true self? Can you really "see" your own soul? We go into these questions in detail. To answer them, you must come to know the nature of the mind (*chitta*) and its activities (*chitta vritti*). You must develop the process of concentrating and focusing the mind (*samyama*), for this is the yogic tool you use to analyze the world and your true nature. In order to develop this tool, you must acquire certain disciplines and attitudes—primarily yama niyama, and *vairagya* (nonattachment). But how? Is this done through practice, willpower, or both? And, what of the obstacles along the way that cloud and obscure the clarity of our vision, such as passion, attachment, fear, and improper conduct? All these matters are discussed in the first chapter, "On Yoga Philosophy."

Asana is the limb of yoga we are all most familiar with. The common understanding is that *asana* means "a posture." But, classically, it is defined as "the seat" or "to sit," and so this term was generally used for a seated yogic position. The Brahma Sutra (a Vedic text on philosophy) refers to asana for meditation. A proper seated posture is necessary to meditate. The idea is that one should be able to stay steady for a long period of time, forgetting about, and undisturbed by, one's own body. How is this accomplished? This is explored in the second chapter, "On Asana and Vinyasa Krama." All the questions in this chapter are asked and answered in the context of vinyasa krama. The primary reference is Ramaswami's *The Complete Book of Vinyasa Yoga*.

The chapter proceeds from the general to the specific. We begin by going into some detail on topics such as breath in asana (a key element in vinyasa krama), bandha in asana, and psychological benefits. Much attention is then given to the subject of proper practice including where to focus the mind. This is followed by discussions of many of the vinyasa krama sequences, following the order of *The Complete Book of Vinyasa Yoga*, and a few specific asanas, with questions ranging from vinyasas of *sarvan-gasana* (shoulder stand) to where to place the feet in *catushpada-pitam* (table pose). The chapter concludes with some additional material on practice.

The third chapter, "On Pranayama," is about yogic breathing techniques. It is said that pranayama is the greatest *tapas* (means of purification). It is pranayama that removes the dross, the impurities, covering the mind, and prepares us for meditation. The relationship between the breath and the life force is an intimate and deep one. In fact, the same word, *prana*, is used for both. We explore this relationship as well as pranayama technique, use of the bandhas, and *kapalabhati* (rapid abdominal breathing), which is technically a *kriya* (cleansing process) but relevant as a preparation for pranayama.

The fourth chapter, "On Meditation," first discusses chanting and *mantra* (a potent word or sound linked to the Divine). Through chanting a mantra, we seek our own link to the Divine. There are many mantras in the Vedas (scriptures) such as the famous Gayatri (mantra on the sun). The *Yoga Sutra* suggests the *pranava* ("OM") for those who believe in God and gives us the method of *japa* (repetition), along with contemplation of the mantra's meaning.

Next, we explore dharana, dhyana, and samadhi, the three processes that are the heart of meditation. We go into some depth on the objects suitable for meditation, such as the breath, *jyotish-mati* (radiant light), and the chakras. Included are a classroom practice for meditation, and a discussion of the difference between Hatha and Raja (royal) yoga. We conclude with a discussion on pratyahara that, although not part of meditation proper, is an important preliminary.

The Raja yogis understood the physiology of the body and the psychology of the mind. The innovations of yogic breathing exercises, exercise of the internal organs through *mudras* (seals) and bandhas, and the positional advantage of inversions were their contributions to keeping the whole body healthy. They also studied the causes of mental ailments and developed attitudinal, dietary and psychological parameters for leading a healthful life. This approach came to be known as *chikitsa krama* (therapeutic methodology), and is the subject of the fifth chapter, "On Yoga Therapy." It is highly relevant during midlife. Chikitsa krama is a wide-ranging subject with as many approaches as there are yoga teachers. We have only included a handful of random questions that came up during our time together, including how much or how little anatomy needs to be studied, and the importance of sarvangasana in therapy.

Much of yoga seems concerned with matters that transcend and are beyond what we normally encounter in life. Is yoga relevant to our daily lives? The last chapter, "On Everyday Matters," touches on issues that are raised by ordinary people leading ordinary lives and asks what yoga has to say about them. Conscience, happiness, despair, religion, memories, conflict, and loss of a loved one are among them. As a bonus, we have been able to include here a few of Ramaswami's personal reminiscences about his teacher, Krishnamacharya.

WHY WAS THIS BOOK WRITTEN, AND FOR WHOM?

We wrote this book to fill a gap in the literature between the beginner's-level introductory asana books and the oftentimes difficult-to-pierce classical Indian commentaries. So much of yoga is learned by the student asking questions of, or even challenging, the teacher and then assimilating the answers. This book is the record of one student's grappling with the concepts, ideas, and practices of yoga, and the assistance, guidance, and insight offered to him by his teacher. Yoga is a vast subject, the questions are without end, and the answers need to be constantly reformulated by each teacher for each student. At best, a book may serve as inspiration to go on and learn more. This book was written in the hope of being just such a stimulus.

This book is for yoga students who have begun to inquire and search after their own souls, who have opened the classic texts and found them bewildering, who have stretched their bodies and met resistance, who have become friends with their breath or at least struck up a relationship with it, who have tried to focus their fickle minds, who have been hurt by life and healed by yoga and now want to help heal others, and for all of us who have no choice but to continually deal with the human condition.

HOW TO USE THIS BOOK

This is not a systematic textbook. It is the record of a conversation. As such, it is more of a companion, perhaps a guide. Ideally, you will have some familiarity with parts or all of the reference texts listed on pages xxix–xxxii, and will read straight through the book. We use a citation style for some material, for example, "YS II,15," to mean "*Yoga Sutras*, Chapter 11, Sutra 15." (A key to the abbreviations of the titles appears on pages xxix–xxxii.)

Many Sanskrit terms are used, for this is the language in which yoga was originally written. We have provided brief definitions whenever the words first appear and occasionally when they reappear in a new context, as well as a glossary/index of Sanskrit terms on pages 238–253, for those unfamiliar with the terms or their derivations. Be aware, however, that many Sanskrit words do not yield to brief translations and a few are virtually untranslatable.

While reading the book straight through may be ideal, it is not usually how we learn and it is certainly not the only approach possible here. You can just as well browse through or jump about from topic to topic, creating your own conversation, because the answers serve are separate independent essays on the various topics. Remember, learning is not always in a straight line. There are some subtle points in yoga, and different ways of thinking. Sometimes going on and coming back, following a zigzag track through the material, is best. What will happen, of course, is that you will begin the process of asking and seeking answers to your own questions. We could wish for no more.

A Note on the Reference Texts

MOST OF THE questions in this book are based on one or more of the following texts. Following their titles are the abbreviations used throughout the book in text citations. Please refer to the bibliography for recommended editions and more information.

Yoga Sutras of Patanjali *(YS)*

This is the most important text on yoga. Patanjali's yoga treatise is written in cryptic statements (*sutras*) and contains four chapters (*padas*). The aphoristic language is of a very high order and his choice of words is extremely precise, making it more like an exquisite set of lecture notes than a book. Because of this, the text must be initially read with a commentary.

For Patanjali, yoga is defined as *samadhi* (concentration). He describes the ultimate goal at the outset, addressing himself to the highly evolved yogi. Having finished with the most evolved, the requirements of the less evolved are taken up in great detail and the means (*sadhana*—"practice") are explained.

There is an authentic commentary on the sutras by the sage Vyasa. Other well-known commentators are: Sankaracharya, Vacaspatimisra, Rajabhoja, and Sadasiva Brahmendra.

Yoga Rahasya of Nathamuni *(YR)*

The *Yoga Rahasya of Nathamuni* is a work by Krishnamacharya, inspired by his devotion to the ninth-century yogi Nathamuni. It's a very important text, useful from all angles, including therapy. This book will give insight into Krishnamacharya's teaching of yoga and also into Vaishnavism, the faith closely followed by Sri Krishnamacharya. It includes many of the teachings Krishnamacharya was famous for, such as adjusting the yoga to fit the individual (*viniyoga*), including his/her stage of life. Special features are yoga for women and yoga for pregnancy.

Hatha Yoga Pradipika *(HYP)*

The *Hatha Yoga Pradipika* of Svatmarama is a classic text, arguably the most authentic and exhaustive work on Hatha yoga. Its four chapters focus on *asanas* (postures), *kumbhaka* (yogic breath control), *mudras* (seals), and *nadanusandhanam* (meditation on a mystical sound). The first three are Hatha yoga and the fourth is supposedly Raja yoga. There is a detailed commentary written in simple Sanskrit by a sage named Brahmananda, which makes it a very useful reference work.

The HYP is the most followed text by Hatha yogis. Sri. T. Krishnamacharya, however, disapproved of some of the mudras, such as *vajroli*, as counterproductive, dangerous, and despicable practices.

Yoga for the Three Stages of Life *(YTSL)*

The three aspects of yoga—as art, as therapy, and as philosophy—are presented in Ramaswami's *Yoga for the Three Stages of Life.* Yoga as an art is appropriate for the young, who need to practice the asanas with all their vinyasas, for growth. As a physical therapy, yoga is well suited for the middle-aged, who need to remain healthy and strong to carry out their responsibilities of family and work. And, as a philosophy, it fits those who have completed their responsibilities and are now entering a time of deep meditation.

The book follows the thought progression of Patanjali, adding material gathered by Ramaswami from his guru, Krishna-macharya. The first chapter is a moving account of the author's long relationship with his teacher. Important asana sequences, pranayama, mantras, and the philosphy of yoga are presented. The book includes a chapter on yoga for women.

The Complete Book of Vinyasa Yoga *(CBVY)*

This is a comprehensive user's manual, by Srivatsa Ramaswami, of the vinyasa krama of asana practice, as Ramaswami learned it from Krishnamacharya. Detailed instructions are given for each vinyasa of ten sequences. Included are the standing, seated, lying, inverted, and meditative pose sequences. *Visesha* (special) vinyasa kramas are also given. The importance of breath in asana is emphasized throughout. And there's a final chapter on the proper way to end a practice. The book is fully illustrated with more than one thousand color photographs.

The Yoga Yajnavalkya *(YY)*

The Yoga Yajnavalkya is an ancient exposition of yoga. Krish-namacharya gave considerable importance to this yoga text. It is quite elaborate, containing several Hatha yoga practices not found in other texts. Of special interest is chapter 4, "On Pranayama" (yogic breath control), which gives a thorough view of the subject, covering techniques ranging from the spiritual to the therapeutic. The book also explains *kundalini* (energy as coiled serpent) in terms of *prana* (the life force) and the *nadis* (pathways), completely demystifying this often confusing concept. The text is written in the form of a conversation between Yajnavalklya and his wife, Gargi. Here yoga is defined as the union of the *jiva* (self) with the *parama* (divine).

Yoga Makaranda (Honey of Yoga) *(YM)*

This was the text written by T. Krishnamacharya in 1934 for the Maharaja of Mysore. A small book explaining the system of vinyasa krama, it is an incomplete work on yoga. The author chose only a few sequences to include as samples.

1

On Yoga Philosophy

INTRODUCTION

YOGA IS TRADITIONALLY considered one of the six orthodox *darsanas* (expositions/philosophies) based on the authority of
the most ancient scriptures, the Vedas. It is a way of life, and consists of a thought process that addresses the most fundamental
questions, such as "Who am I?" or, more specifically, "What constitutes the self?" It not only answers these philosophical questions,
but also gives the necessary practices/exercises for the body and
mind to be in a fit condition to ponder deeply over them. This system of yoga, propounded by Patanjali and based on the scriptural
authority, is known as Raja (royal) yoga. Just as a king is looked
upon by his subjects as a beacon of light, Raja yoga is called "yoga
of light" or "enlightenment," with the word *raja* literally meaning
"light." In four chapters consisting of close to two hundred sutras
(pithy aphorisms), the *Yoga Sutras of Patanjali* address several
questions, such as the nature of mental pain; the cause of such pain;
the actual removal of pain; and, finally, the means for using yoga
to remove that pain completely and permanently. As yoga requires
sensitivity and concentration, the sutras also address the question

of physical and mental practices, which logically and definitely lead to a "one-pointed" mind—a mind that can remain focused on one object continually without being distracted by alien thought or ideas. By sadhana, a habitually distracted mind is transformed into one that becomes habitually one-pointed.

Yoga is neither dogmatic nor a free-thinking philosophy. It is very well structured. It takes into account the different temperaments of earnest people, and suggests different methods to obtain the necessary mental faculty of one-pointedness. Hatha yoga, especially its postures and breathing exercises, is considered to be a stepping-stone toward the exercises of the mind, as stipulated in Raj yoga. Every Hatha yoga practitioner would therefore do well to study Raja yoga, to know the ultimate goal of yoga—*kailvalya* (freedom), which is achieved only by understanding the true nature of one's self. Yoga, Samkhya, and Vedanta are three philosophies considered to result in complete and everlasting freedom. There are some basic differences among the three sibling philosophies, but absolute and irrevocable freedom is the ultimate goal.

Over the centuries, several commentaries have been written about the *Yoga Sutras of Patanjali*. Several contemporary writers have written extensive elucidations of the sutras. Because their thought process is somewhat unusual although still profoundly logical, it is usually necessary to study them with a teacher at first.

YAMA NIYAMA

DAVID: The text (YR I,19) says yamas (don'ts) and niyamas (dos) are to be practiced first and, once these are practiced, then the prescribed asanas are to be practiced. But how? Are they to be accomplished through willpower? Or, do they arise naturally, as siddhis, through correct practice? Or is it some of both? And, how do we make yama niyama part of our daily practice?

RAMASWAMI: First let us see what are yamas and niyamas. They are the first *angas* (parts) of the eight limbs of yoga, or Ashtanga yoga, perhaps the most comprehensive of all yoga systems in vogue. One can say that the yamas and niyamas are the legs on which the whole edifice of yoga stands—without these there can be no meaningful yoga practice possible.

Yama comes from the root *yam*, meaning "to control." Control of what? Control of one's relationship with the external world. The yamas are:

- *Ahimsa* (nonviolence)—don't harm others. Your relationship with all beings in the universe is governed by ahimsa. You should practice nonviolence in your relationship with all beings, without exception. According to the texts, you should not harbor violent thoughts, nor speak in a way that hurts or physically harms others.
- *Satya* (truthfulness)—don't lie. Truthfulness should govern your communication with others.
- *Asteya* (noncovetousness)—don't steal or covet others' possessions.
- *Brahmacharya* (celibacy/faithfulness)—don't transgress the institution of marriage.
- *Aparigraha* (nonaccumulation)—do not pursue wealth and power.

Why are these controls necessary? Because without them, you will constantly be distracted by the elements of the external world and all of your time is going to be consumed by fights, deception, and other corrupting thought processes, the very mental activities the yogi wants to eschew to begin with. These are not for ordinary people, but a serious yogi can make little progress without them.

The niyamas are also five in number. These are the controls to

3

be sustained all the time, indicated by the prefix *ni-*. The yamas are the "don'ts," whereas these are the "dos." They are:

- *Saucha* (cleanliness)—cleanliness of the body and purity of mind.
- *Santosha* (contentment)—contentment all the time, irrespective of the situation.
- *Tapas* (austerity)—restraining the senses. My teacher would say that moderation in food and speech are the hallmarks of this yogic trait.
- *Swadhyaya* (study of scriptures)—study of all relevant yogic and other spiritual texts, which helps the yogi to understand yoga better.
- *Ishvarapranidhana* (worship of the Lord)—doing one's duties diligently as an offering to God.

There is no violent yogi. Nor is there one who utters falsehood. Bandit yogis are nonexistent. Philandering and yoga do not mix. Avarice also is not a yogic trait. Yogis have clean minds and bodies. Contentment is the hallmark of a yogi. Moderation is a yogic virtue. A yogi is a scholar as well. All that the yogi does, he does so with a sense of loving offering to God.

All the yama niyamas are to be practiced, or may I say adopted, by the yogi. They are necessary prerequisites and required to be developed as a habit. Patanjali has used a number of sutras to drive home their importance.

Each one of us is born with different tendencies. Some people are basically angry, some are habitual liars, some have sexual obsessions. But all these tendencies are not conducive to yoga practice, especially the higher ones. So a person who has taken to yoga as a spiritual mission, after acquiring some conviction that yoga will lead the way to kaivalya, will have to spend time and effort to cultivate these traits of nonviolence, and so on. Otherwise an angry young man, without deliberate attention and effort, will end up an angry old man, despite all other efforts. In fact the sage Vyasa, in his commentary on *Yoga Sutras*, compares the yogi who has taken to yoga and transgresses the yama niyamas to a dog who eats its own vomit.

Patanjali advises us to constantly remember that any such transgression is motivated by greed, anger, delusion, and other nonyogic traits. Patanjali also warns that if you do not take necessary corrective action to reorient your conduct, you will become full of misery and spiritual ignorance, which will lead to endless births and deaths.

Many yogis advise their students to ponder at the end of the day all the nonyogic activities they did on that day and take a vow not to repeat them. Constant remembrance of these traits will slowly transform the mind of the practitioner to one that is more yogic, that is, nonviolent, peaceful, and so on. There are some excellent prayers that drive home this point.

DAVID: You mention constant remembrance as a technique for acquiring yama niyama. Doesn't Patanjali also suggest pratipaksa bhavana (thinking of opposites) as a method?

RAMASWAMI: Certainly. Then the first step is to review your actions vis-à-vis *himsa* (violence) and other nonyogic tendencies. That is, to remember or recollect, on a periodic basis, your actions—and to analyze them. If you find that your actions are not according to the yama niyamas, you should consider yourself to be no better than the "dog-eating-its-vomit" example given by Vyasa. These nonyogic activities—be they mild, moderate, or fierce—are prompted by greed, anger, and infatuation. Unless you correct yourself by eschewing these tendencies, you will fall into the old trap of pain and ignorance, with no end in sight. So every now and then, you should reflect on your actions, whether contemplated or caused by others to commit, or actuated by yourself, then think of the *pratipaksha* (opposite), so that you can return to the normal yogic behavior of ahimsa and the other yama niyama. The whole point is that there has to be a conscious effort, at least in the initial stages. Thereafter, habitually, you become a nonviolent, truthful, nonpossessive person. I may mention at this juncture the daily ritual done at dawn as part of daily ablutions in Sun worship, which contains the following prayer:

6

> May the Sun [*surya*], the deity of anger [*manyu*], and the senses that induce anger in me protect me from the sins committed due to anger. Whatever sins I have committed with my mind, with words, with my hands, with my feet, with my stomach [eating unwholesome and non*satwic* food], and with my generative organs may the deity of night destroy them. All the sins I have committed in this birth and those in previous births I throw into the pure glow of the Sun

I used to ask when I was young whether this will encourage everyone to do sinful acts and then pray for forgiveness in this manner daily. Elders used to say that repeated remembrance in this manner will work on the mind and, in a short period of time, one becomes a *punyatma* (virtuous person), and will glow and shun forbidden actions.

Commitment to the yama niyamas and constant effort over a period of time create the necessary *samskaras* (habits). I have discussed this in some length in my book, *Yoga for the Three Stages of Life*, page 91.

VAIRAGYA

DAVID: Is *vairagya* (nonattachment) something we can practice? Is it accomplished by willpower, does it come about as a result of correct practice, or is it a combination of both? I see, in the comment to YR I, 22, that there are two kinds of vairagya. In the early stages, we have to make a conscious effort, and this is called *aparavairagya* [*apara* meaning "lower"]. And, in YS I,16 it states that it is knowledge of *purusha* (self) that leads to the higher vairagya, known as *paravairagya*.

RAMASWAMI: What does the word *vairagya* mean? *Raga* is 7
derived from the root *anj*, or *ranj*, meaning "to stick to something like a paste." So *raga* means "attachment." One is unable to disassociate oneself from the object. The prefix *vi* here indicates "without"; "without attachment" will be *viraga*. And the quality or capacity to remain without attachment is *vairagya* (*viragasya bhavah vairagyam*).

Aparavairagya has to be practiced. You see aparavairagya and paravairagya mentioned in the first chapter [of the *Yoga Sutras*], which is intended for the highest yogi. The yama niyamas are meant for the mid-level Ashtanga yogi, and some for the lower Kriya (yoga of action) yogi. There is a well-laid-out procedure for practicing and developing aparavairagya, and I have explained it in my book [*Yoga for the Three Stages of Life*, pages 51–52]. Paravairagya is possible only after the realization of the true nature of the self, or purusha. At that stage, the paravairagya occurs naturally. If I get the job of the president of the United States of America, will I care or even think about the delivery-boy job I had just before, in Pizza Hut? So when you realize your self, and have a mind that is totally transformed by constant thinking or meditation on the true nature of this self, you will naturally develop paravairagya.

PURUSHA

DAVID: In *Yoga for the Three Stages of Life*, page 49, you talk about the chitta (mind) directly experiencing the purusha. I didn't think this was possible. I thought that we could only experience an object that is part of *prakriti* (nature). I thought the idea was to purify the mind, to make it pure satwa (fit for subtler yogic practices as meditation). Then the buddhi (intelligence) will be a reflection of the purusha. It is this reflection which we "see" or experience. Is this incorrect?

8   RAMASWAMI: All *my* life, I am the subject and the various things in the observed universe are the objects, whether beings or nonbeings. When we sit across a table and talk to each other, so far as I am concerned, you are the object and I am the subject. What is the process by which I see you? Light falls on you, and some of the reflected light enters my eyes and hits the retina. The retina converts the light to impulses that travel through the nerves to the brain. Don't yawn, please; listen to me a little longer. According to scientists, the brain interprets the signals and thus I am able to see.

Let us go a little further. The signals have gone into me. The brain interprets them and this happens within me, within my brain. But how do I see you outside of me? The brain projects (*vritti*) the signals after coordinating with other signals and reconstructing them. So when I see you, I see my mind's projection of you, inside my brain, but appearing as if the image of you is outside of me. This takes place not in physical space (*bhuta akasa*) but in mental space (*chitta akasa*). So when I see you, I only see my mind's projection of you. So is the case with all other objects around me.

Not only that. The mind also projects me seeing you. Obviously, when I see you, I also feel that I am sitting at the table across from you. Though I do not see my full physical body, I am aware that I am talking to you, just as I feel now. I am also vaguely aware of the space around me. Furthermore, when the signals come from you, my mind also interprets the signals, intellectually and emotionally, and I have a composite experience while talking to you. So my experience consists of my sitting, seeing and listening to you through my eyes and ears, and having a composite experience, continually.

So what do we have now? I started by sitting and talking to you. Now I realize that I am the observer of *my* mental projection, which consists of the experience I had to start with. I am not just the physical person sitting and talking, but the one that is aware of the changing projections of the mind. That is, I am the principle that constantly observes what is happening in the mental plane. In the mental space, the vritti consists of me (the sixty-five-year-old me) using my senses, my eyes and ears, and experiencing a person (object) like you. So the subject is my "self," which is pure awareness and the object is my *chitta vritti*. The chitta vritti, or the object, will consist of the empirical self, the senses, and the objects of experience. This is called *triputi*, or the three-factored. Patanjali calls them *grahita* (subject), *grahana* (senses), and *grahya* (objects).

If this is settled, then we can also observe that my chitta vrittis are not confined to the external world. I may observe objects and misinterpret them, in which case the vritti is called *viparyaya vritti* (erroneous projection). Or I can close my eyes and dream (day or night) in which case it is called *vikalpa vritti*. Or my mind can be completely blank, as in sleep. Or I can keep myself amused by recollecting past experiences. So the understanding that what I experience is only mental projections and "I" am the observer, which can be known from the scriptures or through a teacher, is the first step. Once this kind of approach appears logical to me (it may take several days or months or years to get used to this thought process) then I will settle down to the understanding that the chitta vrittis are the objects. I will also know the difference between the sixty-seven-year-old "I" and the observer "I." I will meditate upon or constantly think about the newly discovered "I" or the subject. Slowly, but surely, when the knowledge that I am pure consciousness and the "now happy, now unhappy" Ramaswami is just an object in the mental space becomes firm, my mind will become established in the self,

9

which is the observer of the vrittis. Ultimately, due to yogic practice, my mind will be without any vrittis and my intellect will tell me that "I" am pure disinterested observer. The yogis call this experience *yougika pratyaksha* (direct perception through yogic means). Adi Sankara (expounder of Advaita philosophy) calls the process *samyak darshana* (perfect or true perception). I think it is a question of semantics to say whether the mind can experience the true self. The mind definitely has to recognize the existence as distinct from the ego, which is also called the pseudo-self. In Vedanta, they call the experiencing of the self *aparoksha anubhuti* (nonindirect experience [i.e., direct perception] of the self. Brahad-Aranyaka Upanishad exhorts that the self is to be seen, heard (from scriptures), meditated upon (*mantavya*), and merged into (*nidhidhyasitavya*).

In *Yoga for the Three Stages of Life*, I have explained that this process has stages. First, this idea about consciousness (*chit*) and the field of experience (chitta) being different is to be recognized. Many people may read it and may dismiss it as uninteresting or incorrect. Those who recognize the logic behind it will start deliberating on it. That is the second stage. In the third stage, the mind is completely transformed and does not waver from the knowledge of the self. This stage, in which the mind is in total *nirodha samadhi*, is the third and final stage. In this, for the mind, there is no experience other than the self. To get to this stage, the mind will have to become completely satwic, and hence the need for all the sadhanas.

There are many examples used to explain the two selves. First is the real self, purusha (the observer), which we have arrived at by regression. The other is the pseudo-self, which everyone is familiar with and with which the mind associates itself. The example of the individual self as a reflection of the purusha is resorted to by Vedantins to explain the one consciousness, or Brahman; and the many individual souls (*jivas*). If we have to reconcile to one Brahman and many jivas on the one hand, and the one Brahman not multiplying itself on the other, we have to explain it. One example they resort to is the one Sun and the many reflections of the Sun in many puddles of water.

I am not sure if I have explained it well, but I am sure there will be more questions. I will try to answer any supplementary questions you may have.

DAVID: The key point in your answer, for me, is what you call "yougika pratyaksha." Through practice of yoga, the mind is without vrittis—I become a purely disinterested observer. Maybe it is a matter of semantics, but it seems this "knowing" that I am my purusha is different than the "knowing" of an object. What I experience is mental projections. Mental projections are vrittis. And, if purusha is not a vritti, how can I experience it? To say "the intellect telling me..." seems different from direct experience. It seems more of a deduction. Am I caught up in the semantics here? Is "the intellect telling me..." considered direct experience, only direct experience of a kind other than the usual one of observing the mental projections?

Is the process we are discussing, the one described in YS III,35? There, in Vyasa's commentary, a conception is formed of purusha as being distinct from experience, and samyama is performed on that conception. By that, knowledge of purusha is gained. But that conception is not purusha. That conception is a vritti. So, there is no direct experience of purusha.

Maybe in this samyama on the concept of purusha, knowledge of purusha is gained in a new way, a way that is not inference and not what we normally call direct experience, but rather what you refer to as direct perception through yogic means. Is that possible?

RAMASWAMI: An Ashtanga yogi who reaches the stage referred in YS III, 35, has traversed a long distance. One has practiced the yama niyamas diligently and has considerably reduced distraction from the external world and personal distracting habits. By asana, one has been able to reduce rajas and thus eliminated the instability of the mind and body. Practice of pranayama was helpful in reducing the tamas, and one's infatuations of worldly objects, laziness, and indiscrimination have been eliminated. One's mind has become satwic, fit for samyamas (focusing of the mind). Thereafter, one has used one's satwic mind to do samyama on several objects, gross and subtle, external and internal. By this, one has obtained direct knowledge of these objects. Predictably, one also has developed vairagya toward these objects and has now come finally to get to know the nature of the self, one's own self.

Until now, explaining the practice and experience has been quite easy. Now how to understand the self that is, itself, the observer? Can we properly explain this? Can the chitta understand the self in the same way it understands other *prakritic* (natural) objects?

In this sutra, an attempt is made by Patanjali to explain what should be done to understand the self. If anything at all is to be done, it should be by the chitta in its pure satwic form. Since it has already mastered the samyama of objects and it has developed vairagya on all of them, it has basically only the self to be known. Vyasa, while explaining this endeavor, mentions the reflection or a concept of purusha, and samyama is done on that. However, if you read the sutra, it may be interpreted as dwelling on the distinction between purusha and chitta (*satwa*). By this contemplation, the yogi will be able to know the nature of the self. How does it work? The yogi contemplates on the distinction as follows: The purusha is *avishayi* (not an object) and it exists for itself (*swartha*). The chitta is a changing object (*pratyaya*) and is experienced (*bhoga*) and is meant for the other (*parartha*), which is the self and not for itself. Thus these two phenomena are distinctly different (*atyanta* [complete] and *asankirna* [separate]). This atyanta asankirna can also be interpreted as very proximate but entirely different. Some scholars give the example of an emulsion: the oil and water are close to each other but do not become homogeneous.

12

So here what do we have? The samyama here is on the dichotomy between these two very look-alike principles. By samyama on the difference, the yogi gets to know the unknown (self) from the known (chitta). His understanding of the self becomes absolute.

The argument that this is not a direct perception is true, but only from the point of view of subject-object relationship. This is a unique situation, which normal words cannot explain, especially using the same language as you use for normal transactions. So the Upanishads say, "How can one know the knower?" Now once the samyama is done on the difference, the chitta gets as much of a perfect understanding of the self as possible. Once the chitta is convinced that, by a process of elimination, it has known the truth about the self, then that exercise is over. That absolute conviction is the key. That is yougika pratyaksha. Then what happens? The chitta loses interest even in that knowledge (that is, experiences vairagya). Now the chitta has known everything that has to be known. Then the last stage of the resolution of the chitta takes place: The chitta, instead of being satwic, slowly reaches a stage in which all the three *gunas* (attributes—satva, rajas, and tamas) reach a state of balance (*samya avastha*). A chitta that has reached this stage will continue to be in the guna-balanced stage and will offer no vritti. This is mentioned in YS III, 55. Again, here the sutra talks about pure state of Purusha and the satwic state of chitta. Here, purusha is *suddha* (pure). It is always pure. It is defined as pure consciousness (YS II, 20). Now, due to this samyama, and the vairagya on this knowledge as well, the chitta reverts to its original *mulaprakritic* (unmanifest origin) state (in which all the gunas are in perfect balance), which is called *samya avasta*. That is what the sutra says. It is a state in which the purusha is suddha and the chitta is *samya* (balanced). And that state is called *kailvalya* (freedom), kailvalya for both the chitta and the purusha, as the last sutra of YS indicates.

13

The understanding of the purusha is unmistakably certain to the yogi. We cannot use the normal connotation of "direct experience" here. In Vedanta also, they use the indirect method. To arrive at the atman, the technique of "not this, not this" (*neti neti*) is used. On that knowledge, when the Vedanti gets into samadhi, it is called *nirvikalpa samadhi* (samadhi without ideation [ideation = the process of creating feelings or imagery]). The means may be indirect, but the knowledge is unambiguous. I feel that understanding an object by samyama, and understanding the self that is itself is the knower, are two different situations. That is why I indicated that we should not concern ourselves much about semantics, but only with the reasoning and the process. I concur with the last sentence of your question.

DAVID: Can we say that, in Vedanta, the self is *sat* (existence), *chit* (consciousness), and *ananda* (bliss), but that in yoga it is only chit, consciousness?

RAMASWAMI: The definition of *satchitananda* implies that the Brahman is the source of existence (*sat*), consciousness (*chit*), and happiness (*ananda*) for the individual being. The more the mind turns toward the self, the more happiness it experiences.

In yoga, we have the purusha described as *drashta*/chit, or consciousness. Furthermore, like the self of Vedanta, it is also considered eternal, as it is said to be *aparinami* (nonchanging). I would say that both sat and chit would apply to yoga's purusha.

PANCHAMAYA MODEL

DAVID: In the Taittiriya Upanishad, we are given a model of the human, the *panchamaya* model consisting of five layers, or sheaths. It begins with the food body, the *annamaya*, and proceeds, layer by layer to the innermost, the *anandamaya* (full of bliss). Each layer lies within the one that precedes it. And, it seems, each is deeper than the one preceding. So, the pranamaya lies within and is subtler than the annamaya. Was this model accepted by Patanjali?

Where is purusha in this model? Is purusha the anandamaya or is purusha the entire model? According to this model, our emotions or deep character traits, which lie in the *vijnanamaya* (intelligence), are somehow deeper (closer to purusha?) than our thoughts, which lie in the *manomaya* (mind space). But, in the yoga sutras, we don't find these distinctions. There, we have our *samskaras* (habits), some of which may be more firmly in place, more deeply rooted, than others. But they could be a habit of thought, or a habit of emotion. Both thoughts and emotions take place in the chitta. So, I don't see this notion of one being "deeper" than the other. And, of course, purusha is separate and distinct from prakriti. No one part of prakriti is "closer" (or "deeper") to purusha than another.

RAMASWAMI: This question will have to be answered from two perspectives. How close are the yoga sutras to this *upanishad vidya* (knowledge)? Then, what is the main difference between Panchamaya Kosa Vidya, which is a Vedantic approach, and the yoga sutras, which is a yogic approach?

The yoga sutras and this upanishad vidya try to indicate that the self is pure consciousness and is the observer, and that everything else that is experienced will be the observed and hence not the self. This upanishad takes the example of a sword kept inside a sheath. This is just an example for us to understand that the self is subtler than the sheath, not necessarily inside spatially. The energy, or *prana*, sheath is subtler than the gross; the mind (*mana*), the intellect (*vignana*), and bliss (*ananda*) sheaths are said to be subtler than the previous ones. Anandamaya is considered jiva (soul or self) by some Vedanta schools, but Advaitins consider it as outside the pure self, as bliss is something that is experienced, and the experiencer is different from the experienced.

15

The yoga sutra model is slightly different, but essentially drives home the same idea that the self is different from what is experienced by it. The yogis call everything that is experienced *chitta vrittis*.

Some Vedantins follow the same approach. When the intellect is active, that is, when one is analyzing or deeply contemplating, it is *buddhivritti*. When the mind is coordinating the senses, it is called *manovritti*. Likewise when one is emotionally involved about oneself (*ahamkara*) then it is called *ahamkaravritti*.

There is however a major difference between yoga and the Upanishads. Yoga recognizes prakriti as the object but purusha as the subject. Prakriti and purusha are different and distinct. But for Vedantins, there is only one principle: that is Brahman/atman, which is pure consciousness. What manifests as prakriti arises out of Brahman, and is not different from it. Per Taittiriya Upanishad (a classic in Vedanta), the created universe arises from Brahman, is sustained by and within Brahman, and dissolves in Brahman.

❧ WILLPOWER ❧

DAVID: How are "will" and "willpower" understood in yoga? Is will just another vritti? Does it always arise from desire or anger? Is the will to live, the so-called survival instinct, identical with *abhinivesa* (fear of death)? Do the will and willpower always come from *kleshas* (mental afflictions)?

RAMASWAMI: Will, or willpower, indicates the energy of an individual to pursue a chosen goal—the goal to acquire something he/she thinks of as desirable or to get rid of something that he/she may consider undesirable. Such a person is *rajasic* (characteristic of energy). People without such willpower, who give up easily, are *tamasic* (characteristic of darkness), or weak.

In yoga, willpower is necessary, and one should also have a goal, the yogic goal, which is kaivalya, freedom. If I have the goal of kaivalya, but I do not have the will to work toward it, I will not succeed. So from the yogic point of view, we should be clear about two things: the correct goal and the will (*sankalpa*) to pursue the correct practices.

If the goal is different, say, becoming a millionaire (or more), or to achieve a high position in life, then also one should be strong willed to achieve that. But, if the goal is not kaivalya, then all the actions of the mind, including the strong will to achieve the goal that is different from kaivalya, will be *klishta* (unfavorable) vrittis or those that will produce further klesas, or pain.

17

✺ TAPAS ✺

DAVID: In YR I, 70, as well as in many of your answers to my questions, the concept of satwic food is mentioned. Is this food that is light? Or food that makes you feel light? And, what of the difference between Eastern and Western diets? Do we still have a concept of satwic food in the West? Does it mean being a vegetarian?

RAMASWAMI: For the beginner, the first aspect of Kriya yoga (yoga of actions) is *tapas*. What is tapas? According to Sadasiva, the author of *Yoga Sudha* (commentary to the *Yoga Sutras*), tapas is the intake of moderate, agreeable, pure food. The food should be satwic. What is satwa? Satwa is lightness of body and enlightenment of the mind. So food that is easily digestible, food that does not excite or clog the *nadis*, is satwic food. *Hatha Yoga Pradipika* and the Bhagavad Gita (Song of Lord Krishna) give a list of satwic food items. Since the subtle part of the food we intake forms our mind, our mind becomes satwic, rajasic, or tamasic depending upon the type of food we take. Hence, considerable importance is given to the food.

When I started teaching yoga several years ago, I was advised not to trouble the sensitivity of students by suggesting lifestyle changes, especially food. But Patanjali says the intake of correct food is absolutely necessary. So, all students will have to ponder over these aspects if they are serious about the practice of yoga. As animal food is considered rajasic and alcohol is considered tamasic, all serious students of yoga should consider the reduction and ultimate elimination of these items from their diet. Even a number of vegetarian food items are non-satwic.

18

SATWIC MIND

DAVID: Can the mind ever be pure satwa? Aren't the other two gunas (rajas and tamas) always present as long as the mind exists?

RAMASWAMI: The chitta is always comprised of the three gunas. What is done by the yogi is to make the satwa the predominant quality, by weakening the other gunas. The other gunas become dormant by these practices; it happens and is strengthened by samskara. When the yogi repeatedly keeps his/her chitta in the satwic mold, it remains predominantly satwic.

Thus we have people who continue to be satwic all their lives. The rajas and tamas are dormant but can come up if the satwa is allowed to weaken over a period of time. That rajas and tamas continue to be present is evident from the fact that, in the ultimate *nirodha* (complete stoppage) stage, all the three gunas are said to achieve samya avastha (the state of balance).

SWADHYAYA

DAVID: Do you understand *swadhyaya* as the study of scriptures and repetition of mantras? What about knowing oneself, or self-knowledge? Is this included under swadhyaya?

RAMASWAMI: *Swadhyaya* is a compound word and also a Vaidic word. *Swadhyaya* was split as *swa* (one's own) + *sakha* (branch [of scriptures]) + *adhyaya* (chanting/study and the resultant expertise) by my guru. It means studying one's own branch of scriptures. My guru gave considerable importance to swadhyaya— chanting, study, and expertise in authentic scriptural texts. Since yoga is considered an ancient science and practice, and considerable reference is given in the scriptures, swadhyaya is an inherent and important part in the development of a yogi. Since yoga, Vedanta (ultimate truth of Vedas, scriptures), and other philosophies of the scriptures help us to understand the nature of the true self, swadhyaya is to be considered an essential element in the sadhana of a yogi. I have dealt with this aspect in my book, *Yoga for the Three Stages of Life* (pages 67–76). There are several important references there to the study of the self. In fact, the ultimate goal of the scriptures is to help you understand the true nature of your self and attain permanent peace.

19

DAVID: Are you saying that when we learn about the self being distinct from the mind, or about the five *mayas* (layers) from the scriptures, then we are gaining a deep understanding of ourselves, and that this is swadhyaya; but that when we go to therapy and untangle our emotional history and better understand our personality, then this is not swadhyaya?

RAMASWAMI: I am not familiar with modern therapy, which will lead one to untangle one's emotional history or better understand one's personality. But this should be good. If you can become more stable, happier, better able to understand why you behave the way you behave, it would certainly help you. But the word *swadhyaya* is used in a traditional sense to mean understanding the true nature of the self. Psychoanalysis does not approach it in that way. In these analyses, the self is not considered pure consciousness, as a mere observer. Since the basic tenets of yoga and these modern approaches are different, it will be difficult to include these analyses and therapy under swadhyaya.

I feel that the interpretation given by my guru for swadhyaya, as the study of one's own scriptures, is the correct one. The bulk of the Vedas consists of hymns, prayers, and rituals dedicated to different gods. Patanjali, while giving the benefit of swadhyaya, says that it will result in the communion with those gods (YS II, 44). Since, in the Upanishads (the source books on Vedanta), the scriptures devote a considerable portion to the understanding of the self, it is also conceded that swadhyaya could mean to study portions of the Vedas that lead to the understanding of the self, which in turn will result in *moksha* (ultimate release). But these are not the objectives of modern analysis, and it may even frown at these concepts and approaches.

For a yogi, analysis is certainly welcome if it helps reduce or eliminate:

- Anger/violence
- Lying, manipulating, gossiping, rumor-mongering
- Coveting/stealing
- Possessiveness/miserliness
- Sexual indulgence/obsession
- Unclean habits
- Habitual depression
- Gluttony
- Dislike for philosophical studies
- Lack of respect for God (Superior Being)

In fact, I mentioned earlier that some repeated reflection on one's negative conduct (for example, anger or violence) on a regular basis will slowly free the mind for better yogic practice and contemplation. One can do the analysis oneself or take the help of others qualified to help, such as one's the teacher. But the word *swadhyaya* has a clear-cut connotation, as explained. It may not be correct to say that swadhyaya includes psychoanalysis and psychotherapy.

❧ SCRIPTURES AND POETRY ❧

DAVID: In answer to one of the chikitsa questions, you spoke of Kriya yoga as the yoga suitable for those who are old or sick and cannot do any asanas. Along with chanting and study of scriptures, you suggested poetry or anything else that would be uplifting. Why would poetry, etc., be considered Kriya yoga? Are they somehow related to *Ishvarapranidhana* (devotion to God)?

Is this related to YS I, 39, where the suggestion is made that anything that brings stability to the mind may be used? (Only, I assume, it needs to be "uplifting.")

When I was young, I used to study mathematics. And, even now, reading some mathematics can quiet my mind and bring stability. Is this what is meant?

RAMASWAMI: I am sorry that my earlier answer was not clear. Usually, in these contexts, I use the term *scriptures* to indicate the Vedas. But in India, these scriptures were memorized and studied by only a small segment of the population. What about the rest of the people?

In the olden days, many works, such as *dharma sastra* (works on *dharma* [law and piety]), *smirtis* (scripture-oriented works), *puranas* (divine stories or god stories), and *itihasas* (great epics, the most famous being *Ramayana* and *Mahabharata*) were all written in verses or poetry. So what I mean by poetry is these kinds of works. Then there were several moral stories and works, such as the Bhagavad Gita (Song of Lord Krishna), *Yoga Vasishta* (Vasishta's Yoga), and others. All these were poems; very few were written then in prose style. Poems helped the author to give vent to his poetic abilities and also help prevent interpolations, to a great extent, as it is more difficult to tamper with poems.

So what I meant by poetry are works that are consistent with the ideas and ideals propounded in the Vedas. These were less terse and thus more easily understandable to the larger population. The purpose of swadhyaya and Isvarapranidhana, in Kriya yoga, is to considerably reduce the mental pain of the practitioner. We must also remember that it will be difficult and inappropriate for the beginner's-level yogi with a heavy heart to attempt some of the yoga practices mentioned in the first chapter, which may I remind you is for the *uttama*, or the highly evolved yogi. The beginner's-level yogi is advised to start on Kriya yoga, mainly because he/she cannot, or is not yet fit to do the *ekatawabhyasa* (practice on one principle) mentioned in YS I, 39.

HAPPINESS AND LOVE

DAVID: You make the point in *Yoga for the Three Stages of Life* that, unlike Mimamsa (a school of philosophy) and Vedanta, yoga is concerned with avoiding pain, not with gaining happiness. This is a disappointment to me, and I think to many students who come to yoga hoping for a happier life. True, to the yogi who is as sensitive as an eyeball, all is suffering. But, though they are ephemeral, do not love and the satisfaction of work well done count for something? What of the notion of bliss? Commentaries on YS I,17 refer to *sananda-dhyana* (meditation on the blissful feeling). And, YS II, 42 states *santosha* (contentment) brings happiness. In addition, on page 126 of YTSL, you mention a positive sense of well-being coming from asana practice and a sense of calm from *pranayama* (yogic breath control). Cannot these be regarded as steps toward happiness? Are they all only measures to reduce pain?

RAMASWAMI: There is considerable sibling rivalry among all the Vedic philosophies, even as they all vouch for the authenticity of the Vedas. Thus we have Mimamsa, or Purva Mimamsa, which exhorts the human being to work toward increasing the happiness, or *ananda*. There are hundreds of rituals that are detailed in the Vedas, all to propitiate different deities. Performance of these rites are considered *dharmic* or *punya karmas* (meritorious activities). These, by and large, will ensure passage to different celestial worlds or heavens after death, with concomitant enjoyment in these worlds. The duration of the stay in these *lokas* (worlds) will depend on the accumulated punyas. After they are exhausted, other sets of ripe karmas, whether meritorious or not, will give their own kind of experience to the individual. However, the incentive for the individual to perform these rituals is the prospect of enjoyment in those worlds, which enjoyment will be much higher and superior to anything an individual can experience in this world. But the Vedanta points out that all the promised happiness is in the future, which is uncertain and impermanent. Furthermore, due to the gradation of happiness experienced, an element of unhappiness is associated with all these by way of comparison, and thus there is nothing like unalloyed bliss in all these heavens. In the Vedanta, there is also considerable discussion about happiness and its gradations. Youth, good conduct, scholarship even while young, perfect senses like sight and hearing, strength, possession of enormous property and riches—all could give maximum happiness to an individual in this world. Yet, a hundred times happier, say the Upanishads, will be the soul in the celestial world. Then the discussion goes on to enunciate worlds where higher and higher levels of happiness can be found. Please refer to page 38 in my book YTSL.

What prompts people to aspire for higher happiness? They are tormented by desire. It is true of all the endeavors for happiness here and hereafter. Quoting the same Upanishad, the Vedantins say

23

that a consummate scholar or wise man is able to achieve the same level of happiness mentioned earlier by not being tormented by such desires (*akama hatasya*). Hence the prescription of desirelessness and correct knowledge of the self gives complete freedom from the restlessness experienced by the person with passionate desires.

24

Mimamsakas and Vedantins talk about happiness and the means of achieving it, whereas Samkhyas and yogis find that a large majority of people, rather than desiring happiness arising out of getting the desired object, would yearn for relief from misery they are experiencing. The relief from *duhkha* (pain) is tantamount to happiness to them. So, to appeal to them, these philosophies start by saying that the duhkha should be eradicated. The Vedantins' dig at the Mimamsakas for their obsession with happiness is matched by the concern of the yogis for those who are in misery. Ultimately, Vedanta (Advaita or nondual), Samkhya, and yoga all prescribe the correct understanding of the nature of one's own self, as pure, nonchanging consciousness leading to the ultimate good.

What is happiness? Is it the result of the fulfillment of desire or the removal of pain?

DAVID: Are you saying that, from the point of view of yoga, love is simply the fulfillment of a desire?

RAMASWAMI: We desire a thing when we know it will give us happiness. Because it gives us happiness, we love it. There may be selfless love or sublime love, but basically the object should have the capacity to give you happiness.

There is an interesting episode in the Brahad-Aranyaka Upanishad. Yagnyavalkya was a great Vedic scholar. For his scholarship and insights, he was sought after by wise men, powerful men, rich men, and many more. He became very rich. He had two wives, Katyayani and Maitreyi.

Toward the last stage of his life, he called his spouses and wanted to make a deal with them. He said he wanted to take *sanyas*, the fourth and final stage of living one's life. He offered to split his enormous wealth between the two wives. Maitreyi asked him whether all the wealth he would give her would make her immortal—implying thereby that what Yagyavalkya was after was immortality. He answered in the negative. In response, she requested him to instruct her on how to attain immortality.

As was his wont, Yagnyavalkya started from the known to make the disciple understand the unknown. He said, "It is not for the sake of the husband, my dear, that he is loved, but for the sake of the wife that he is loved by the wife. Likewise, it is not for the sake of the wife, my dear, that she is loved, but for the sake of the husband that she is loved by the husband." He went on to add that love toward children, wealth, clan, heavens, deities is similar. It is not for the sake of all that all is loved, but for one's own sake that all is loved. So who am I, for whose happiness all this is loved? Therefore, the conclusion was that "The self, my dear Maitreyi, should be realized—it should be heard from the scriptures, reflected upon repeatedly, and meditated on. By the realization of the self, my dear, through hearing, reflection, and meditation all is known."

So we love beings and objects that we think will give us happiness. To obtain that happiness, we endeavor to get and retain that beloved object. But, depending upon the quality of the mind, happiness is achieved by different kinds of objects. According to ancient smritis, the human goal is fourfold: *dharma* (piety), *artha* (possessions, power), *kama* (sensual gratification), and *moksha* (release). People who are predominantly satwic (the characteristic of light and clarity) derive happiness by doing dharmic work, whereas rajasic people love possessions and power because that will give them happiness. Tamas-infested people will love objects that give happiness due to the excitement of senses. Each group

25

❧ SAMYAMA ❧

DAVID: In chapter III of YS, why does Patanjali use the word *samyama* instead of *samadhi*?

RAMASWAMI: Sometimes you may be able to get into samadhi on one object (*sampragnata samadhi*) easily. Getting to complete samadhi could be a process for the beginning Ashtanga yogi. He/she starts with dharana (concentration), wherein there is a great attempt to keep focused on one object. The ability to keep trying to be focused on one object is itself an accomplishment. Once this is done then, continuing in the practice, if the fledgling yogi is able to remain with the object uninterruptedly all through the meditation period, it will be *dhyana* (meditation), and then samadhi (absorption) in the same object will be the end of this series of contemplation.

Yoga and Samkhya (a Vedic philosophy) expect the practitioner to do this set of internal practice not with one aspect of prakriti, but all the twenty-four *tatwas* (eternal principles) and then finally the twenty-fifth *tatwa*, the purusha. There are many people who master all three on one object, but are not able to transfer the same concentration to other objects. So when they start the practice on a new object, they soon lapse into samadhi on the earlier object, the one they had already mastered samadhi on. Here Patanjali says, inter alia, that starting dharana on one object and ending the session in samadhi on another object will not be samyama. So *samyama* is a word used to describe the process in which the dharana, dhyana, and samadhi are all on the same object. Patanjali says *trayam* (all three: dharana, dhyana, and samadhi) *ekatra* (on one object) *samyama* (is samyama).

DAVID: Once samyama is acquired, is the idea to run through the tatwas, from gross to subtle, eliminating them one by one, as not belonging to the self? Or, is this the procedure from Samkhya? If so, what is the method of the *Yoga Sutras*? And, if we believe in Isvara (God) do we skip the tatwas and go directly to him?

RAMASWAMI: When "what is" is camouflaged by "what is not," then it becomes necessary to analyze everything to distinguish (*viveka*) between the two. Then it may become possible to discard "what is not" so that what remains is just "what is." The Samkhyas say that the cycle of samsara (the endless cycle of death and rebirth) can be cut asunder only by knowing the self. And since, for the ordinary individual, the self is mixed up with many a nonself, one has to carefully study and analyze everything—self and nonself—before eliminating the nonself. So they insist that the only way (*eikanthika*), and also the sure way (*aatyantika*), is to know all tatwas: the one self and the twenty-four nonselves.

So by a process of elimination, one starts from the gross and proceeds slowly, deliberately, to understand each and every one of the twenty-four nonself tatwas, and discards each of them. This will not be possible without deep self-analysis. When the subject goes through this process, however, in the end he/she is sure of what is not the self. He/she becomes convinced that the twenty-four principles—from the gross elements (*bhutas*), to the senses, the ego, the intellect, and the "unmanifest" (*mula prakriti*)—are not the self. The person's conviction is so complete (*apariseshaha*) that he/she is able to remain steadfast in the state of knowledge that he/she is not the possessor of any part of prakriti, be it worldly objects, the body, or the senses (*na mey*). The second conviction is the total negation of the common feeling of "I" associated with his/her body (*na asmi*), the sheer feeling of "I exist" (*asmita*). And third, the association of agency with the body/mind complex, which we normally identify as ourselves, is also completely eliminated from his/her mind.

While the Samkhyas say that one should thoroughly understand the twenty-five tatwas to achieve kaivalya, it is not possible without acquiring the capacity for unwavering concentration and commitment. This is what is achieved by the yogic step-by-step approach. Yogis give the means of developing a mind that has the capability to unwaveringly focus on these subtle principles. Toward that end, yoga also suggests Ishvarapranidhana as an alternative means. So the idea is to first get the mental capability of yogic samyama, and then to run through the principles from the gross, through the undifferentiated set of principles, then the intellectual ones, and finally the unmanifest prakriti. And every time the yogi is able to know one principle or group of principles thoroughly and is convinced that it (they) is (are) nonself, he/she discards attachment to that tatwa as being the nonself, and proceeds further.

The third philosophy of truth, the Vedanta, also proclaims a similar approach. Here the ultimate principle, the truth, which exists forever, conscious and undifferentiated, is called Brahman/ atman. Here also, the approach is to get an empirical knowledge of the ultimate reality through the texts (Sastras, Vedas) first. Then, the aspirant broods over or contemplate the principle of nonself and discards it as "not this, not this" (neti neti), that is, as not the Brahman/atman. When everything that is nonself is thus eliminated, the truth dawns in his/her mind clearly. A very vivid example of this approach can be seen in Taittiriya Upanishad, Bhrugur Valli, in which there is the episode of Varuna (Vedic god of rain) and his son, Bhrugu. In this the student, step by step, understands that the body, then the bio-energy (*prana*), the mind, the intellect, and the ego do not constitute the self.

Where does Ishwara come in? Samkhyas want the aspirant to use only his/her intellect to understand all the tatwas. They neither believe in nor have any use for Isvara. Yogis, going by the popular emotive means of devotion, suggest that going to Isvara will solve the problem. But, in truth, worship of Isvara will give the aspirant the mental capability to analyze all the tatwas and dichotomize the self from the nonself. Here Ishvara is potentially a repository of all knowledge, including of the self. The Vedantins also suggest *bhakti* (worship) of the Lord who is no different than the Brahman, gives the aspirant what he/she wants.

So if he/she approached the Lord with a wish list of name, fame, wealth, and a superior afterlife, the devotee would get it. But only the one who prays to the Lord for release—the final release (moksha)—gets it. The lesson here is that one can try different means, but salvation comes ultimately from one's effort. Even to seek the Lord's grace needs individual effort. And the Lord gives the aspirant the necessary capability. The famous Gayatri (prayer Vedic mantra on the Sun) is for stimulating the intellect, so that the aspirant will know the ultimate truth. One of the common wishes children in this part of India—south India— are encouraged to pray for is a "good mind."

VIKALPA

DAVID: Are infinity and eternity examples of *vikalpa* (imagination)? If we think of these as qualities of God, can they be considered *aklishta* (favorable) vrittis?

RAMASWAMI: Some vikalpa vrittis are *klishta* (unfavorable) from the point of view of spiritual progress and peace), and some are favorable. If we consider firmly that infinity and eternity are qualities of God as enunciated by scriptures, then chitta vrittis on these lines will be considered aklishta vrittis. The methods of meditating upon the Lord as Brahman, having the qualities mentioned, are contained in several Upanishads, such as the Taittiriya Upanishad. The method of giving a form, attributes, names (*mantras*) are all aklishta vikalpa vrittis. When meditation on these is done regularly, one can get into samadhi on the imagined attribute, in which case it is called *savikalpa samadhi*.

Infinity and eternity, per se, are not vikalpas. They, along with awareness, define what Brahman, or ultimate reality, is. Our normal minds cannot grasp infinity or eternity because we know of nothing in real experience that is infinite or eternal. According to scientists, even the universe, wherein objects could be as far apart as millions of light years (the Sun is said to be just about eight light minutes afar), is said to be limited but unbounded. Further the universe is also not eternal, in the sense of something that is not changing. A thing that undergoes change but exists forever is not considered eternal (*satya*, or truth) by Vedic scholars. Only God or Brahman is considered eternal and infinite. So if we try to fathom eternity and infinity by using the observed universe, it is just impossible. However Upanishads talk of the universe as emanating from Brahman (God), as being sustained by it, and as eventually merging into it, only to reemerge. So the meditation upon the universe as a manifestation of God or Brahman is vikalpa, but such mental activity will be aklishta vritti, because the meditator goes into *savikalpa* (with ideation) samadhi with the ultimate reality. It is said that when the meditator is able to go beyond the limitations of savikalpa meditation and merge with the ultimate reality (Brahman or God), that state is called nirvikalpa samadhi.

With the mind's limitations, it is not possible to know infinity and eternity. The Brahman is defined as pure consciousness (*gnana*), which is eternal (*satya*, nonchanging). Because it encompasses and permeates the universe, it is also said to be infinite (*ananta*).

According to Advaita Vedantins, the same pure consciousness that is eternal is the core of all beings. If the individual can grasp that and can go into samadhi with his/her own soul, then he/she knows Brahman.

That Brahman or God is infinite is brought out in an interesting story told by Saivites (worshippers of Siva). The trinity of Brahma (creator), Vishnu (sustainer), and Siva (destroyer) were

in a discussion. Siva was said to be infinite. Vishnu and Brahma
challenged this, and said that they could find out the beginning
and end of Siva. If that was done, it would be proved that Siva cannot be said to be Infinite. Siva spread himself as a beam of light
that extended up and down the universe. Brahma flew up in his
swan vehicle, while Vishnu took his boar incarnation and moved
downward. After a long time, Vishnu and Brahma returned to the
meeting point. Then Vishnu said truthfully that he was not able
to find the end of Siva's beam of light. Brahma said that he was able
to see the other end, and brought with him the fragrant aloe vera
plant to vouch for him. It was a lie, and Siva became furious with
Brahma. He punished Brahma, and also directed that none should
worship Brahma; hence there are no temples for Brahma. And the
plant/flower aloe vera also was banned from being used as an offering to the Lord.

DAVID: Since infinity and eternity arise out of the meaning of
words and are not real things, why are they not examples of
vikalpa?

RAMASWAMI: No. Here we are using the words, however
imperfect they may be, to explain a reality.

I presume that the words *eternity* and *infinity* are the translation
of the Sanskrit words *satya* and *ananta*, when used with reference
to Brahman/God/Isvara. These words signify a reality, the absolute
reality, and not vikalpas. According to the Upanishads, the definition (*swarupa lakshana*) of Brahman is satya (truth, existence,
or eternity), gnana (pure consciousness), and ananta (infinity).
Satya indicates a thing that exists eternally or that which never
undergoes a change (*aparinami*). So what this word signifies is a
thing that is beyond time. The word *anantha* means that which has
not been limited by another, or that which is beyond space. Gnana
is pure consciousness. So the definition of Brahma according to

this statement (Satyam Gnanam Anantham Brahma) is that Brahman is pure consciousness that is beyond time and space. This is the classic definition of Brahman from Taittiriya Upanishad.

Even though *infinity* and *eternity* are words that may not indicate anything specific that we know of in the universe, as a definition they help us to understand the *swarupa*, or nature of Brahman. Here again one can see that since we can know finality and limitation of all objects, by distinguishing Brahman from these (not limited by time or space), we are able to form a first impression about Brahman. Though the learner has not experienced Brahman as a yogi would have, he/she still has the first clue about something that exists. To explain something that is beyond our experience with words having limited reach, but that is still real, one has to resort to words that point to it only in an indirect way. The Upanishad also expresses the difficulty of explaining and understanding this reality. "The words trying to define it return without defining it (Brahman). The mind trying to know it also returns without grasping it (Brahman)."

With respect to objects in the universe, there is nothing which the mind can comprehend that is eternal (in the sense of non-changing), nor anything beyond space (infinite). But these words can point to an entity that is real, and still beyond the restrictions of time and space with which the mind is familiar.

How does one give the definition (or attributes) of infinity and eternity to Brahman? Because it is said that the enormous but limited universe was born out of it, is sustained by (in) it, and eventually resolves into it. The universe that we know is limited (however enormous it may be) and transient, because it merges back into its source. The universe is therefore finite and transient. Brahman, which is its source, is therefore considered infinite and eternal. Thus we may conceive the Brahman from what we know of the known universe.

✣ MAITRI ✣

DAVID: In the practice of YS I, 33, it is suggested that if we practice friendliness toward those who are contented, compassion toward those who are suffering, appreciation toward the virtuous, and avoidance of those who are evil, it can have a steadying effect on the mind. Need we be careful that friendliness (*maitri*) might lead to attachment to people? That would be a klesha. And, similarly, should we be wary that joy (*mudita*) might lead to or become passion?

RAMASWAMI: This is one of the methods suggested for steadiness of mind, especially for those who are gregarious, compassionate, appreciative, noncombative. The yogi is in such a satwic stage that he/she will not get passionate or attached to someone, as we normally understand the term. I have seen several saints, or *sadhus*, who will talk with friendliness, be compassionate when we suffer, or are appreciative of any dharmic activity that we may do. There is always an aura of warmth, compassion, or encouragement when we meet them. But they live like the drop of water on a lotus leaf or duck skin—close but never attached.

✣ SVASA-PRASVASA ✣

DAVID: In YS I, 31, the symptoms of a disturbed mind are given. One of them is *svasa-prasvasa*, which is usually described as the breath being disturbed. But, doesn't *svasa* simply mean "inhale" and *prasvasa* simply mean "exhale"? And, in that case, isn't Patanjali simply referring to normal breathing? That is, it would appear normal breathing would be regarded as a symptom of a distracted mind. This seems to be what Vyasa is suggesting in his commentary.

RAMASWAMI: Patanjali uses the term svasa-prasvasa to indicate the whole activity of breathing in two different places, one in

YS I, 31 as you have indicated, and also while explaining pranayama in YS II, 49. Our breathing can be classified as under (a) voluntary control, (b) involuntary control but can be brought under control, and (c) involuntary control but cannot be brought under voluntary control. In pranayama, we deliberately bring the breath under voluntary control. During normal breathing, the breath is in involuntary control mode, but can be brought under control mode by will. But in the context referred to in YS I, 31, the breath is under involuntary control but cannot be brought under voluntary control. Here, the concomitant symptom, svasa-prasvasa, should be read with other symptoms such as *duhkha* (internal pain), *daurmanasya* (weak mind), and *angamejayatva* (trembling). There will not be normal breathing with the mind experiencing duhkha and body trembling. So one should infer that normal breathing is not indicated in sutra YS I, 31, but uncontrollable or heavy breathing. Hence Patanjali suggests a regular practice of long exhalation in the sutra I, 34 to create the samskara of calmness in the mind of the yogi, so that whenever the mind relapses into a stage of *vikshepa* (*disturbance*), manifested as duhkha or other symptoms (YS I, 31), it can quickly recover to the state of normalcy and proceed to attain *ekagrata* (one-pointedness).

35

❧ ON KLESHAS ❧

Moha

DAVID: Does *moha* (delusion) differ from *avidya* (misconception)?

RAMASWAMI: According to Samkhyas, *moha* is a manifestation of tamas in the mind. It is infatuation. *Avidya* is wrong understanding. But with reasoning, a person with avidya gets vidya. But a person with moha gets attached to an object while completely overlooking all the faults of the object. Samkhyas refer to different gradations of tamas. They say that there are eight types of moha, ten types of *mahamoha* (great delusion), eighteen types of tamisra (another name for intense delusion) and then *andhatamisra* (highest level of delusion), all manifestations of tamas.

Ego

DAVID: A question on ego: I think of three meanings for the word in English. The first is "pride." When someone is boastful, or showing off, we say he/she has a big ego. The second use of *ego* is for who we think we are by association: I am the body, I am the mind, and so on. And third, it stands for the simple statement "I exist." Are all these covered by the term *asmita?* I can see how the first can be reduced through humility and modesty. I can see how the second can be eliminated through viveka, knowing who we truly are. But, the feeling of "I exist"—can this really be eliminated, or is it with us as long as we are alive?

RAMASWAMI: Samkhyas refer to three afflictions that the *tatvagnani* (one who knows the twenty-five principles) overcomes. The three afflictions are *mey* (mine), *aham* (I), and *asmi* (I exist). All the three afflictions are removed in the gnani because he/she knows the true nature of the self, which is mere observer. "Mine" is an attachment experienced by everyone. Aham is the feeling of "I," or ego as you have put it: I am poor, I am rich, I am the greatest yoga teacher. Then, even for the devout gnani, the nagging feelings "I exist in this body"—Vedantins call these *mamata, ahanta,* and *asmita.* According to Patanjali's sutras, as long as avidya (ignorance) about the true nature of the real self persists, the most immediate cognition of asmita comes into being.

It is true that the asmita will be there until death. But it is only so for the nonyogi. The yogi who has reached the state of kaivalya would have transcended even the "I exist" feeling. Since chitta has reached a stage of nirodha, his/her mind will be in nirbija samadhi and he/she will be oblivious to everything including his/her own existence, as if in a trance. Asmita, as we can see, is not always manifesting. In deep sleep, in coma, and in samadhi, it is dormant or absent. So, according to yogis, the only way to remove the wrong identification of the self is to know, by samadhi, the correct nature of the self. While practices like modesty and other agreeable qualities will make one less boastful and less conceited, total eradication is possible only by correct perception (samyak darshana) of the true nature of self.

37

Raga

DAVID: Is it right to say that desire is included under *raga* (attachment) as one of the kleshas? Then we practice Kriya yoga to weaken the klesha and Ashtanga yoga to annihilate it. But, can I ever truly eliminate desire, as long as I am alive? Must I simply accept my desires, work hard to achieve them, and just not be attached to the rewards (Isvarapranidana) or results of my efforts?

RAMASWAMI: I think the English words *desire* and *attachment* are related. I desire a thing because of the perception that it will give me pleasure or happiness. I get attached to it because it gives me pleasure or happiness.

To merely act to achieve what you want so as to satisfy your desires, and to then say "I am offering the results to the Lord," it is incongruous. You are acting to satisfy your desires, which may or may not be dharmic. So if someone does prohibited actions, satisfies his/her desires, and says that he/she offers the results to the Lord, it is just not acceptable. He/she will certainly suffer the consequences of vicious activities here or hereafter. The Lord's words direct one to do those duties that are prescribed (*vidhi*) and shun those that are prohibited (*nishedha*). Furthermore, I do not think it is possible to desire a thing, enjoy it, and then forego the attachment to the object.

Ishvarapranidhana in yoga occurs in three different places. I have dealt with the three aspects of Ishvarapranidhana in *Yoga for the Three Stages of Life* (pages 76–78). As a Kriya yogi, one has to observe Isvarapranidhana along with tapas and swadhyaya, both of which will ensure that one will not do acts that are *adharmic* (antiyoga). Tapas, which in the broader sense means the control of senses, will not permit one to do anything and everything to get what one desires. Here Isvarapranidhana, per the commentators, is worship of the Lord. In the next higher Ashtanga yoga stage, again with the other yama niyamas, Isvarapranidhana is included. Here it means the offering of the results of your actions to the Lord. But one's actions are themselves governed by the other yama niyamas, such as nonviolence, truthfulness, and so on. In effect I have no complete freedom to do what it takes to satisfy my desire and then surrender to the Lord, or surrender my attachments to the Lord.

There is an interesting prayer from the *Mahabharata*. Many people recite it in the morning, which is controversial. (Because Duryodhana was not a pious person, it could mean that whatever evil deeds he did were per the directions of the Lord within. However for pious people it is very good prayer.) It is a prayer by Duryodhana, the king of the Kauravas, who usurped the kingdom of their cousins, the Pandavas. The prayer runs like this:

> *I know what is right [dharma], but I have no inclination to do it.*
> *I know what is wrong [adharma] but I have no inclination not to do it.*
> *So, whosoever Lord resides in me and directs me,*
> *I do according to his directions.*

On one hand, it may be construed as a prayer for beseeching the indwelling Lord to direct the subject on proper lines. However, many others consider it as the justification of a wicked person to

put the responsibility on the Lord for his own adharmic trans-
gressions. Here, the approach should be to progressively reduce
attachment and aversion to objects. This is achieved by the practice of Kriya yoga.

There is a verse in *Thirumandiram*, a very old book, highly
revered by Tamilians in South India. It reads like this:

39

Root out desire, root out desire,
Even to be with the Lord, root out desire
More the desires, more the sorrows,
When more and more desires are given up, more and more the
   bliss will accrue

Another quote from the *Mahabharata*, a favorite among yogis is:

All the comforts [sukha] that acquisition of worldly objects
   may give,
All the great comforts one gets by attaining celestial worlds,
Equal not even just a sixteenth part of the smug comfort
One gets by renunciation of the thirst for pleasure

DAVID: What of those desires that are dharmic? I'm thinking
of family and *abhasya* (practice). We work hard (within the limits of yama niyama) to support our family. But we cannot control
what comes of our efforts. We must be comfortable with whatever
rewards we receive. Similarly, what of our desire to practice yoga?
Again, we must do our practice without expectation of result. Both
are Isvarapranidana. But, on the other hand, we are working
always to reduce raga. So, there seems to be a conflict here. Is this
the problem raised in YR II,38, where Nathamuni states that
householders cannot achieve the *yogangas* (limbs of yoga)?

RAMASWAMI: What is dharma? The word *dharma* comes
from the root *dhru*, "to support." The word *dharani* also comes

from the same root, and dharani means "Earth" because it supports all things on Earth. *Dharana* also comes from the same root. It means holding on to the object of contemplation. That is, the mind supports the object without allowing it's falling off or forgetting. So what is dharma? In Sanskrit, dharma is defined as *"dharate uddharyate va iti dharmah"*: those actions that support and uplift one. So our actions are dharmic if they are wholesome, uplift us, and help in preventing us from falling down. And all societies and communities define dharmic actions. We may say yama niyama and other practices of yoga are dharmic activities so far as a yogi is concerned. This means what is dharmic for a normal being may not be so for a yogi. And dharma also varies under different circumstances. That is, for a Brahmachari, the one in the first stages of life, celibacy is a dharma; so is the case with the one in the fourth ashrama, sanyasa. But for a *grahastha* (a family person), it is not the dharma. Likewise, possessions and taking compensation for rightful work are dharma for a grahastha but they are taboo for the other two ashramis mentioned. In another example, rajadharma (what the king or the government can do for the general welfare and uplifting of the community) could be adharma for an individual. A king can confine a criminal or even kill him, but for an individual to do likewise is adharma.

The Vedas and the subsequently written Dharma Shastras (dharma texts) extensively deal with dharma in all its variations. Basically, dharmic actions are classified as vidhi, or those actions that are to be compulsorily done. While doing these karmas prevents you from falling down, they, per se, do not uplift you to higher worlds such as *swarga* (heaven). Not doing the vidhi karmas is adharma by omission.

There are activities that are called *kamya*, dharmic actions with a motive behind them, such as attaining heaven in the life beyond. These activities, when performed correctly with a lot of sacrifice, will uplift the individual to greater worlds of bliss. These

40

are not obligatory duties, and failing to do them does not bring any demerit. However, there are those who will still do these activities because the discipline involved has the potential to keep the mind pure, without desire for the results promised in the Vedas, such as going to heaven. Here, the satwic or dharmic activity is done for the sake of the activity alone and not for the results.

It is customary to start all Vedic activities with a *sankalpa* (a resolution or statement of purpose). While a person who does these activities with the desire for the results specifically states the purpose at the time of samkalpa, the desireless person will do them with the resolution that the results of his/her dharmic action should go to the Lord (Isvarapranidhana), thus indicating he/she does not want the results of the dharmic activity, but does it only for the purification it brings to his/her mind.

So, all activities aimed toward the reduction of raga are dharmic activities of a yogi. A rajasic person should endeavor to reduce it by appropriate yogic practices and yoga dharmas. For example, asanas tend to reduce rajas. But the word *raga* is usually used for infatuation and slavish desire to objects of the world, not for satwic or dharmic desires. In fact the Advaitins (nondual Vedantins), who want to develop extreme vairagya, also talk of intense desire as a basic requirement for moksha. What is that desire? It is the intense desire for release from the clutches of samsara or the cycle of births and deaths (*mumukshatwa*).

Can a householder be a yogi, too? Yes, the first- and perhaps the second-level yogis can be householders. There is intense discussion about a householder, or even a former householder, being able to reach the Vedantin's moksha or the yogi's kaivalya. Take the case of *aparigraha*, not receiving compensation for lawful service rendered, and saving for a rainy day. A householder with responsibilities toward the family members will have to earn and save. There are so many dharmas a yogi has to follow. My teacher used to say that in this modern time of *kali yuga* (the age of strife), it

41

is almost impossible to follow all the yogic dharmas, especially for householders. While everyone practicing yoga should endeavor to follow them, some of the yogic principles may even conflict with having a family.

There are those who assert that lifelong celibacy (for those with a natural celibate tendency) is a necessary condition for spiritual freedom. Some say that naishtika Brahmacharya—lifelong, flawless celibacy—correctly interprets the word *Brahmacharya*. This will naturally exclude all householders. But there are those who interpret Brahmacharya to suit householders by saying that sex within the institution of wedlock is acceptable.

My guru would say that the only dharma a yogi will be able to follow completely in modern times (Kali yuga or the age of strife) is Brahmacharya, which he would interpret as nontransgression of wedding vows. According to him, lifelong celibacy is a wish and almost everyone who takes this vow fails. His advice would be to follow the rules or dharmas for each stage of life and live a life of contentment and total surrender to the Lord. So, for a grahastha it is almost impossible to follow the yogic dharmas in toto. Still, constant endeavor to diligently practice dharma and constant bhakti (devotion) to the Lord (Isvarapranidhana) will take one far on the path of yoga.

So it may be good to note that all activities of yogi should be dharmic. And a person who does not want to be tied to the results of his/her actions, like heaven, etc., may well surrender the results of his/her satwic or dharmic action to the Lord.

It should be noted as a corollary that adharmic activities should not be performed. There is no escape from the law of karma that will visit the *kartha* (doer) of adharma at the appropriate time. You cannot shortchange the Lord with adharma.

DAVID: Is it all right to have a passion for practice? Should we say that it is all right in so far as our practice is reducing rajas and tamas, then it is dharmic? But, if our practice becomes an addiction, then it is raga, a klesha?

RAMASWAMI: If we keep in mind the ultimate goal of yoga, which is kaivalya, and consider all the steps mentioned in classical yoga as a means to that end, then we will not get passionately attached to one practice, like asana, and the pleasures arising out of it. There is considerable logic in the sequencing of the eight steps in Ashtanga yoga (classical yoga). In yoga, the approach is to make the mind one-pointed and to contemplate on the nature of the self, so that kaivalya is reached. The yamas help the yogi to reduce the outward-looking tendencies of his/her mind and reduce the scope of possible conflicts and attachment to the external world. The niyamas are a set of personal habits that will help the yogi to be less and less self-centered. Asanas remove the distractions to the yogi, such as diseases or unsteadiness, that are caused by the body. When the yogi has to meditate and contemplate, he/she does not want the body to be a source of distraction. He/she would like to "forget the body," or be oblivious to the body while in meditation, and this requires perfection in a seated pose. So, if one focuses on the point of kaivalya, the purpose of asana practice is to overcome this "body feeling" and not be carried away by the "body-beauty" feeling, which leads to the attachment or to the addiction you have mentioned. Pranayama clears the mind of cobwebs of tamas, and pratyahara helps to withdraw the senses from their respective objects. Then the yogi is in a condition to proceed with the internal practices, such as samyama, ending hopefully in kaivalya.

If I do asana practice without the ultimate goal in mind, I am likely, inevitably, to be attracted by the beautiful postures my body can take and the great healthful feeling these asana practices give. But if I know the ultimate goal, I will not rest with these intermediate levels of achievements. Patanjali would like the yogi to guard against being overwhelmed by the ecstasy of *siddhis* (accomplishments). This applies as well to asana siddhi.

43

Many of the people who have come to yoga and stopped with asana practice are those who have mastered their body through several other disciplines, say, gymnastics, dance, or other physical exercises, in which the perfection of the body is the end. A true yogi will not feel satisfied with asana siddhi, and will not stop until kaivalya of the self is achieved.

My guru was a great Hatha yogi. But he did not stop with practice of asanas and pranayama alone. His routine would include meditation on the Lord, study of the texts, and teaching and contemplation on the ultimate goal of yoga.

DAVID: A friend of mine is grieving over the loss of his mother. A very powerful emotional experience. But, this comes about through the attachment he felt for his mother. And, attachment, raga, is given as one of the kleshas to be weakened. Is this really possible? Would the true yogi really feel no grief over such a loss? Would he have no attachment toward his own family?

RAMASWAMI: Lord Shiva ordained that Adisesha, the serpent king, should incarnate as a human being and prepare a text for Sanskrit grammar. Adisesha was born in the world as Patanjali, to a pious woman named Gonika. Patanjali renounced family life after getting permission from his mother to do penance, intense samadhi, and watch the dance of Shiva to prepare for writing the monumental work called *Mahabhashya*. He also would write two other treatises: one for yoga, the *Yoga Sutras*, and the other, *Charaka Samhita*, a text for Ayurveda. When he went out to start his spiritual journey, he assured his mother that he would see her any time she wanted to see him. Gonika, much later, decided to see him once before her death, and Patanjali, a great yogi, appeared before his mother to be with her at the time of her death. One of the wishes of all parents in olden India was to die in the lap of their offspring, and Patanjali fulfilled this last wish of his mother.

A similar story is told of Adi Sankara, the expounder of the

44

Advaita system of philosophy based on the Vedas. At the age of about eight years, he went to a river to take an early morning bath and was mauled by an alligator. When his mother cried for help to save her son, Sankara said that the only way he would survive was for him to renounce family life forever and become a *sanyasin* (one who renunciates). His mother agreed and the alligator, so the story goes, let go its deadly hold. Sankara then took sanyas and, while taking leave of his mother, promised her that he would come to her at any time she wanted to see him.

45

You can see from these stories it is not that the yogis and sanyasins do not love their mother, but they had their own mission to fulfill which was not possible if they were family men. A yogi is not a misanthrope. He/she has sublime feelings, including compassion (*karuna*), happiness (*mudita*), and friendliness (*maitri*). What he/she sees is that our normal way of life of attachment and dislike toward objects and beings is due to ignorance of the true nature of the self, and this attachment leads to misery. In their utmost compassion toward all beings, they would urge everyone to see the misery of life, here and hereafter, and to endeavor to transcend the ignorance about the nature of their own selves and achieve kaivalya as a means to a permanent end to cycles of birth and death and concomitant misery.

Yet he/she is not attached, if that is what the word *raga* means. Patanjali and Sankara loved their mothers, but also realized that death was just the end part of the process of life and accepted the reality with equanimity.

Another story, from the life of Buddha, might be of interest. Once, a young mother with the dead body of her infant son came to the Buddha and begged him to use his occult powers to revive her son. Buddha agreed, but asked her to get some sesame seeds from a household that had not seen any death in the family. Soon the mother realized the futility of her desire and accepted the reality of life and the other side of the coin, death.

Thoughts and memories of the dear ones linger long after they are gone. One may grieve briefly and remember with warmth the good thoughts of the departed soul. Intense raga leads to intense misery after the object is lost or the being to whom one is attached is gone. But sublime love transcends all unhappy feelings, including grief.

46

Abhinivesa

DAVID: *Abhinivesa* is a vasana, isn't it?

RAMASWAMI: If abhinivesa is considered to be, as many experts explain, fear of death, then it can be treated as a vasana, the idea being that the fear of death is inherent, even for the newborn. Avidya is the mother of all klesas, of which abhinivesa is one of the offspring. But if you broaden the definition and consider abhinivesa to mean fear in general, a klesa that afflicts most people most of the time, your purpose then becomes to find a way to overcome that fear definitely and permanently. So from practical point of view, consideration of abhinivesa as a klesa, as misery, is more useful than dealing with it as vasana.

Burnt Seeds

DAVID: Do the kleshas always exist in one's mind? Or, are they gone totally in the state of kaivalya? In Vyasa's commentary on YS II, 4, he introduces the "fifth state" of the kleshas, the burnt seed. The kleshas may be brought to this state by Kriya yoga. Then, while they still exist, they lose their power of producing action. For how can a burnt seed germinate?

Later, we learn that Astanga yoga produces *viveka khyati* (power of discrimination), which annihilates avidya. And, so all the kleshas would be annihilated, too. When kaivalya is reached, and the gunas have returned to their original balanced state, the kleshas would no longer exist. Is this the case, or would the kleshas still exist in their burnt seed state?

RAMASWAMI: For a plant to be created, apart from the seed several other ingredients are required. Soil, water, sunshine are some. If any one of the necessary conditions does not exist, the event does not take place. For a future birth to take place, there should be a bundle of unripe karmas (karmasaya), then ignorance (avidya), and its offspring, such as asmita. If no karmas remain there cannot be a new life, as some philosophies, such as Nyaya, would suggest. But Avidya is the more potent cause: as long as it is there, it will propel the individual to act and accumulate karmas, which when unused would necessarily be stored as karmasaya. So if we can make the klesas impotent, then there can be no motivation or no motivating force to propel the karmasayas to seek a new life. The example of a burnt seed is just an example. Vyasa is trying to state that, just as a burnt seed cannot produce an offspring, avidya is incapable of acting in the case of the liberated soul. We should read it as, "Just as a burnt seed cannot become a plant, so when avidya is annihilated no further life will fructify."

VASANA AND SAMSKARA

DAVID: What is the difference between vasana and samskara? Does *vasana* refer to latent impressions from past lives and *samskara* to mental habits acquired in this lifetime? Already when we are born, some things bring pleasure, others pain. Does our sense of what brings pleasure and what brings pain come from our vasanas?

RAMASWAMI: Vasana indicates that which resides latently. It is the knowledge derived from the impressions left on the mind by past actions, done here in this birth or previous births. One classic example of vasana is the knowledge one gets, at the time of death, about the characteristics required to function in a future birth.

How does a human being function as a worm in the future birth? Because he carries the vasana of a worm, which he was in some previous birth in the chain of innumerable births before.

Samskara is the habit formed by doing an action repeatedly, so that the individual functions in a particular groove or habit. The samskara can be from this birth or even from previous births. Why is one of a pair of twins calm and the other agitated, even at the time of birth? It is said to be due to the samskara from some previous *janma* (birth). The chitta is said to be the remainder (or the residue) of samskaras: *"Samskara sesham hi chittam"* (Man is a creature of his habits). A person who acts in one way for a long time will continue to function in the same way. A pious person continues to be pious because his/her mind is full of samskaras of piety. Changes can be brought about by willful, sustained action. A person who is full of anger samskaras will be angry. But by conscious effort, he/she can replace the anger samskaras by samskaras of calmness. This is called *parinama* (transformation). When actions are changed repeatedly they leave new samskaras, replacing old dissimilar samskaras.

In the final stage, by conscious repeated yoga practice of *nirodha* (stoppage), the yogi replaces the *vythana* (outgoing) samskaras of the chitta with samskaras of nirodha.

DAVID: Are the samskaras and vasanas related to each other in the following way: If I have a samskara, the repeated action of the habit leaves a latent impression (vasana). If I have a samskara of anger or piety, then when that samskara is not active, is it latent (vasana)?

And conversely, when I have a latency (vasana) and this becomes active can it not create a habit (samskara)? That is, can I not have a vasana of anger or piety?

RAMASWAMI: The word *samskara* is derived from the root *kru*, "to do," with the prefix *sum* indicating "totality." Samskara is the result of repeated action—the impressions left by repeated similar action. A well-known example often given is as follows: Between two villages that are sparsely populated, there is a meadow. When people walk on the meadow at different places, the footprints are not discernable. But over a time, people tend to walk along the shortest distance, circumventing such obstacles as elevated areas or ponds or rough, rocky areas. Over a period of time, there wears a footpath created by people taking the same route. Thereafter, almost everyone tends to walk along the same footpath, created by themselves. The path is samskara. Once the path is created, people tend to go by the same path.

49

As a young man, I used to be angry and abusive; I would get things done my own way by using force, verbal or physical. Over a period of time as I grow up, this tendency gets strengthened in me (samskara), and I use the same tactics, even when I am older, because that is my samskara, my habit, my beaten track.

My mind is nothing but such samskaras, just habits. The way I express myself, the awkward way I write English, are all part of my samskaras. Can this be changed? Yes, samskaras can be changed by learning to practice deliberately opposite actions that, over a period of time, will become new samskaras replacing old samskaras. That is also the crux of yoga practice. Change in food habits, exercise, thought processes are all susceptible to change by yoga. You have new yogic samskaras in place of old, distracted, nonyogic Samskaras. This change of one's samskaras is the key to success in yoga.

The word *vasana* is derived from the root *vas*, "to reside." Impressions from old experiences remaining hidden in our citta are vasanas. I learned how to ride a bike when I was five years old. I have not ridden a bicycle in the last fifty years. Still, if there is an opportunity, I will be able to ride it. It is the vasana. Normally, vasanas are considered deeper and they can remain for a long time, even through several births. If I am born as an eagle in my next birth, the vasanas to function as an eagle are already ingrained in me because during the succession of innumerable lives (which cycle has had no beginning), before this present life, I would have spent lifetimes as an eagle, and those impressions are ingrained deep in my subtle body. Hence, when the opportunity arises, I will have the ability to function as an eagle. Both samskara and vasanas are action related. But vasanas are a lot more subtle.

50

A childhood musical prodigy, or a child saint such as Sankara, is born with the latent impressions of music or yoga from their previous births. We use the word *vasana* (or *purva janma vasana*) in such cases, rather than *samskara*.

✢ SVABHAVA ✢

DAVID: What is the concept of svabhava? How does it relate to our vasanas? Our samskaras?

RAMASWAMI: *Svabhava* means "one's nature" (*sva* = one's own; *bhava* = nature). When we say "the svabhava of a dog is to bite," we refer to the nature of the species, or its vasana. Svabhava is innate. When we say that the svabhava of a particular person is nobility, we refer to the person's samskara, his/her natural (customary, not necessarily innate) behavior. We sometimes use the word *svabhava* to refer to the conduct of a person. "He has a good svabhava" means that the person is good-natured.

✢ KARMA ✢

DAVID: In YS II, 13, 14, one of the fruits of karma is our experience of pleasure and pain. Does this mean our karma will determine what, for us, gives pleasure and what gives pain? Does it mean our karma will determine whether our life is a pleasant and happy experience or a painful one? Of course, for the yogi, all of life's experiences are seen as painful but, this comes from viveka, doesn't it? For the yogi, this doesn't come from his/her karma.

RAMASWAMI: Yes. The YS II, 14 clearly indicates that *punya* (meritorious karma), will lead to sukha, or happy experience (*hlada*); and that *apunya* (despicable acts), will result in the opposite, or pain (*paritapa*). But the bundle of karmas that fructify to give a birth is by and large a mixed bag. We experience both sukha and duhkha in a particular life. Some experience more duhkha because of the higher ratio of apunya deeds that fructify in that seen birth (*drishta janma*). The karma bundle also keeps changing (within the limits imposed by the particular kind of janma) depending on the intensity of the karmas done in the present janma. The stories of Nahusha and Nandikeswara exemplify this. However, whatever the yogi does is such that it does not add to the karma bundle, as for normal beings. This is so because, due to his/her knowledge of the self, he/she has no motivating impulse for experiencing the results of his/her karma. And what the yogi does will fall neither in the bad karma nor good karma categories and so will yield no pain or pleasure here or hereafter.

DAVID: In the West, we think DNA determines much of our physical and mental makeup, including much of our personality. In the East, karma is thought of in much the same way. To what extent would you say these two concepts are the same or different?

RAMASWAMI: Karma determines which genes I will acquire in the new birth, the genes of a rat or a royal family member or a diabetic. Genes explain why I behave in this way, why I am a healthy or unhealthy. Karma theory explains how I got these genes in the first place.

KARMASAYA AND VASANA

DAVID: Are karmasaya and vasana related? When we do an action and its karma does not come to fruition, it remains as karmasaya. Isn't this a latency and so a vasana? In *Yoga for the Three Stages of Life*, on page 82, you use the phrase "karma vasana." Is this the same as karmasaya?

RAMASWAMI: Commentators on the *Yoga Sutras* have used the words *karmasaya* and *vasana* (or *karma vasana*) to indicate different aspects. Karmasaya are actions that have been accumulated but that have not borne fruit for want of the right conditions. *Karmasaya* means "stored actions." Supposing I have done karmas, the results of which can be experienced in the form of a species other than human being, then they cannot fructify during this birth. At the time of death, if a dominant karma is one that can give results through the body of, say, a dog, then all the karmas that can fructify in this particular kind of birth will join the main karma to give the incumbent the experiences in a particular lifespan of a dog. But how does the individual get the necessary natural tendency to act like a dog? This is provided by the vasana, or the memory the individual has of dog's behavior from some previous births as a dog. How did he/she get to act like a dog in his/her previous janma as a dog? Again, it is from the previous vasana. This cycle of births and deaths is *anadi* (beginning as less). So Karmasayas are stored actions waiting to give experiences (happy or unhappy) and vasanas are memories that help us to function in a particular *jathi* (species).

SUBTLE BODY

DAVID: We don't know what happens after death. So, this question may not be answerable. I will ask it anyway. Our purusha is unchanging, eternal, pure. It survives death. In rebirth, it returns.

52

This same purusha is now associated with a new body, a new mind. But this new mind has vasanas from past lives of the purusha. How can this be? The vasanas are part of prakriti. The mind, as part of prakriti, does not survive death. Yet somehow these vasanas "travel" along with the purusha and reappear in the new mind. What is going on here?

RAMASWAMI: This question is not answerable because we do not remember what happened before our previous passing away. But the Sastras (scriptures) go into considerable detail and explaining what they say is not that difficult.

There are three classes of prakritic evolution we have to consider here. There is a body called the subtle body (*sukshma sarira*). Then, there is the *mata-pitruja sarira* (the embryo, the body to be born out of the parents), whose various parts are hardly discernable. That is the second body.

The embryo slowly takes space (*akasa*) for itself, accumulates the gross elements of earth (solidity), water (the various fluids in the body), air, and also fire in the form of heat required to maintain life, through the mother's umbilicus. This body slowly evolves into the gross body, the *sthula sarira*, made up of hair, blood, muscles, nerves, bones, marrow, and so on. It is said that of these, from the mother is derived hair, blood, and muscle tissues, whereas from the father come nerves, bones, and marrow. Finally, the full-term fetus is given birth as a grown being with a subtle body. Then the body given by parents acts as a template and fills with the gross elements of the universe, forming, in the third place, the gross body.

The gross bodies repeatedly get destroyed (in death). Further, the dead body if buried, as is the custom in certain communities, becomes part of earth. The same occurs when the bodies are thrown into the valleys, as some communities do, where they are eaten by jackals and vultures. Or they are turned into ashes when burned, following the custom in certain communities. After death, the subtle body is not destroyed but, propelled by its bundle of *dharmic* (righteous) and *adharmic* (sinful) actions, traverses on with the purusha.

At the time of the beginning of evolution, the subtle body is created (based on the previous karmas, which have no beginning) individually, to each purusha. It is capable of traversing through the entire universe, and is capable of remaining until the final evolution (or until kaivalya is attained, in the case of an accomplished yogi). The subtle body is made of eighteen of the aspects of prakriti: intellect, ego, mind, five senses, five instruments of action, and the five tanmatras (irreducible aspects of sound, light, and so on). These carry the characteristics of the three gunas: happiness, pain, and delusion. This subtle body, after the death, leaves the gross body and together with the purusha attains a new body, propelled by the collection of karmas (karmasaya). It is like an actor who takes a new role after completing his portrayal of a character in a play.

The subtle body is capable of identifying completely with a new body, forgetting the old body with which it was associated. How can we explain it? In our own experience, in dreams, our mind identifies totally with a new body created in the dream, the dream self, completely dissociating with body of the dreamer. And it happens over and over again.

This is based on slokas (verses) 38 to 41 of the *Samkhya Karika* (text on Samkhya philosophy). Samkhya is the theoretical basis for yoga. There are several other texts, which explain graphically the transmigration of the self with the subtle body.

❧ TANMATRA ❧

David: Can you help me understand the tanmatras? What is meant when the Samkhya philosophy calls these "the subtle forms of the knowables"? Are the tanmatras involved in the subtle perceptions of the senses called *vishayavati* (relating to objects) in YS I, 35?

RAMASWAMI: *Tanmatra* is a compound word, *tat + matra. Tat* means "that" and *matra* means "merely" or "by itself." So *tanmatra* means "merely that" or "that alone." The tanmatras are terms used by Samkhyas to indicate the basic elements of objects, which can be grasped by the senses. Thus we have *rupa-tanmatra*, which is light (particle) alone. Likewise we have *sabda-tanmatra, gandha-tanmatra, sparsa-tanmatra*, and *rasa-tanmatra*, which are respectively basic elements of sound, smell, touch, and taste.

According to Samkhyas, the evolution is multistaged. The prakriti is made of the three gunas: satwa, rajas, and tamas. All the gunas are in a state of equilibrium (*samya-avasta*) in *mulaprakriti.* At the time of the beginning of evolution, the first stage is the ascendancy of one guna over the other gunas. The first stage is the ascendancy of satwa. From this disequilibrium, the *mahat-tatwa* (the universal intellect) is said to evolve. From that, rajas becomes predominant and we have the *ahamkara* (ego principle) evolving out of it. From the satwic aspect of ahamkara evolve the mind, the five *gnanendriyas* (senses) and the five *karmendriyas* (organs of action). From the tamasic aspect of Ahamkara evolve the five tanmatras. From the five tanmatras evolve the five *bhutas*: space, wind, light, taste, and smell (see also *Yoga for the Three Stages of Life*, page 84).

What are the knowables? Those that can be grasped by the senses are knowables— objects that can be heard, felt, seen, tasted, and/or smelled. We do not see the objects as they are. The sound waves strike the eardrum and, from that sensation, the mind re-creates the object within the mind. Likewise, light particles strike our retina, and in similar fashion the senses "grasp" objects. So it can be seen that these subtle elements of sound and others, called *tanmatras*, actually make it possible to experience the external world.

The vishayavati pravritti mentioned in YS I, 35 refers to the

55

experience the yogi gets by focusing on different spots within the body that will give divine experiences. For instance, it is said that if you can focus on the middle of the eyebrows, at the top of the bridge of the nose, one experiences "divine" smell. The word *vishaya* refers to those kinds of experiences in the occult practices of yoga. This sutra says that, by doing the practices mentioned in the yoga texts, experiences such as the one mentioned take place.

DAVID: Are the tanmatras real physical objects or something subtler? Is the sound tanmatra the smallest possible sound wave that can strike the eardrum and allow the mind to re-create the sensation of sound? Is the light tanmatra the same as what physicists call the smallest unit of light, the photon? Is it the same as a photon striking the retina?

RAMASWAMI: According to the *Yoga Sutras*, the tanmatras are subtle and are classified as Avisesha (nonspecific). They are not gross and cannot be perceived by the senses. What we experience are the visesha, or gross aspects, of the five elements, which create the sensations. Only yogis, therefore, can experience tanmatras, and only in a state of samadhi, the *sampragnata samadhi*.

✿ TIME ✿

DAVID: Can you help me understand YS III, 52, *ksanatatkramayoh samyamat vivekajam jnanam*, which says that by doing samyama moment by moment on the distinction between self and intellect, knowledge of the self takes place? How is it that, by understanding moment and sequence, we can acquire viveka? One seems connected to time and the other to purusha, our true self.

RAMASWAMI: Some aver that the fourth chapter in YS is an addendum. Some believe that whatever Patanjali has to say is complete with the third chapter. In fact this sutra, coming almost at the end of the chapter, comes after a sutra in which Patanjali talks about kaivalya (*Tat vaitagyadapi dosha bijakshaye kaivalyam* [From dispassion the seed of fault is destroyed. That is freedom]). So we have to look at this sutra a little more carefully.

This is a sutra in which Patanjali talks about samyama on time, or more particularly about the basic unit of time that he calls *kshana*, and which can be translated as moment. According to these philosophers, time is sequence of moments. If all the moments in the sequence are the same, then there is no change. So even the subtlest change can be known by concentrating upon each moment and on the sequence of moments. The yogi is able to distinguish the subtlest changes. Normally we do not have that capability. The yogi has developed a keen mind with which he/she can do such profound contemplation.

What is the relevance of this sutra at the end of the philosophical discourse? Right through, the thrust has been to emphasize that normally one is not able to distinguish between chit (consciousness) and chitta (mind). Once the yogi has developed the capability to concentrate intently, to observe momentary changes, he/she will be able to see the difference between chit and chitta. One is nonchanging and the other, changing. By such a close observation of the two (satwa and purusha) he/she finds that in the chitta, change takes place, whereas in the purusha, there is no change. This observation takes place moment after moment in the chitta of the yogi doing samyama. This is not possible for the ordinary mind because it is not able to distinguish between two successive moments. So this power of the yogi to watch each and every moment and see a succession of moments involving change in one case and no change in the other case, leads to the discriminative knowledge between the self and the nonself.

57

❧ TURIYA ❧

DAVID: I've encountered the word *turiya* in some of the Upanishads, whereas the *Yoga Sutras* use the term *samadhi*. Where does the idea of turiya come from? Can turiya be related to samadhi? More generally, I have encountered the names of several yogic states now, can you elucidate the differences among: turiya;, *asamprajnata samadhi* (samadhi without object), the so-called fourth kind of pranayama mentioned in YS II, 51; and *kevala kumbhaka* (breath-holding only) spoken of in the *Hatha Yoga Pradipika*. Or, are these really referring to the same state of mind?

None of these states is the same as kaivalya, are they? (Although it sounds like turiya might be.)

RAMASWAMI: These terms are used in different contexts to indicate the same or similar states. Asampragnyata samadhi indicates a state of samadhi in which the chitta is in samadhi but without an object. If, on the other hand, there is an object with which the chitta is in samadhi, perfect knowledge of the object is obtained (sampragnyata samadhi). Likewise with the terms *nirbija* (without seed) samadhi as opposed to *sabija* (with seed) samadhi. If you want to indicate the state of the mind in which the chitta rejects any object for samadhi, it is called nirodha (complete stoppage). This is so because in the state of nirodha the chitta habitually refuses to entertain any other stimulus/activity. The chitta is completely satisfied, as one would decline a piece of candy when the stomach is full. All these different terms are used contextually. Yoga uses the term *kaivalya* to mean a state of being alone, which is translated in English as "freedom" by many people.

But different philosophies use different terms sometimes. Vedanta uses the term *moksha*, or "release," as the ultimate goal. And, *nirvikalpa samadhi* to indicate a state of mind where there is no ideation of Brahman or the ultimate reality, as opposed to savikalpa samadhi, which would indicate the knowledge of Brahman as the source of the manifest universe. Some Vedanta texts call this the fourth state: if we accept that our consciousness has three known states: waking, dreaming, and sleeping; then the fourth state, which is beyond these three, is the turiya state. Normally, we do not encounter this state at all. Only a Vedantin who attains the wisdom of the nature of the self, and also recognizes that it and the Brahman are one and the same, is able to reach this stage. So we have turiya, nirvikalpa samadhi, and moksha as terms describing the same ultimate state, per Vedanta. Sometimes Vedantins also use the term *kaivalya* to describe the same state.

59

The real question is whether all the final states are identical. Is the yogi's kaivalya the same as Vedantin's moksha or the Bhakti yogi's *sayujya* (merger with the Lord)?

The goal of all these philosophies appears to be the same—the escape from the cycle of rebirth and death—and they would exhort every human being to make use of the present life to achieve this goal or at least work toward this goal. They would say that by the perfect perception (*samyak darsana*) of the reality of the nature of the self, the mind becomes completely and permanently satisfied. In such a state, there is no further desire to satisfy the permanently satisfied mind, and there will then be no further participation in the cycle of samsara. The Vedantin will assert that in the state of moksha or turiya, the subject never returns to be born (*na punh avartate*). So says the yogi of his/her kaivalya.

But the difference lies in the perception of the reality. While yoga says that the individual soul is pure, nonchanging consciousness, the objective world is different from it and is real. The Vedantins will ask the question of why the two distinctly different principles, individual purusha and the prakriti, came together to begin with. Is there another third principle that is responsible for this? These questions are not satisfactorily answered by yoga— say the Vedantins—and the belief is that, if the philosophy leaves a few questions hanging, then it may not produce the same ultimate satisfaction in the subject and the mind may not settle down. Such a mind will continue seeking a satisfactory permanent answer, and may not reach the ultimate goal yogis talk about.

By stating that there is only one principle, pure consciousness (Brahman), and that the evolution (real or apparent, that is another question) takes place from it and not from another independent entity called prakriti (as the Samkhyas and yogis assert), Vedantins overcome the problem stated earlier. So the Vedantin will say that the self is pure consciousness, as the yogis say, but the individual consciousness and the supreme consciousness are one and the same. Since, according to Vedantins, only this knowledge, which alone is correct, will give ultimate satisfaction, this understanding becomes necessary to achieve moksha or turiya.

We can say that both are similar, in that the mind is totally satisfied. Since imperfect knowledge will lead to confusion later on, we have to acknowledge the difference in these states.

✼ TWICE BORN ✼

DAVID: What is the meaning of the phrase "twice born," which occurs in many old Vedic texts? Does this refer to the idea that when we obtain viveka, it is like being born again?

RAMASWAMI: The human birth is the first birth. One is born again by knowing the nature of oneself, by studying the scriptures. Hence, a realized person is twice born. But the word *dwija* (*dwi* = twice, *ja* = born) is given to those who have been initiated into the study of the Vedas and spend their lifetime studying, teaching, and doing the necessary practices for salvation as mentioned in the scriptures.

2

On Asana
and Vinyasa Krama

INTRODUCTION

ASANA MEANS TO sit. A seated posture is considered asana
in yoga parlance. However, over a period of time, several hundreds
of standing postures have also come to be considered as asanas,
provided they meet certain criteria—the posture should be comfortable and steady.

Vinyasa krama is an art form of yoga practice. In this ancient
system, several postures are done in sequences, and the breath and
mind also come into play. All the movements connecting various
postures are done with slow, smooth, *ujjayi* (throat-control)
breathing, and the inhalation and exhalation synchronize respectively with the expansive and contracting movements. The mind
is required to closely follow the breath and in this way the "yoga,"
or yoking of the mind with the body, is achieved with the breath
acting as the harness. Breath awareness, smooth breathing, and
flowing movements all done in unison make yoga asana practice
a very joyful experience.

The use of breath and the mind's focus on the breath, unique to the
system of vinyasa krama, is based on the instructions of Patanjali in

the *Yoga Sutras*. So in the Raja yoga method of asana practice, the parameters to be considered are steadiness of postures and movements, a high level of comfort, synchronized breathing, and continuous breath mindfulness. There are more than one thousand vinyasas (variations and movements); about ten to eleven sequences of them are currently in vogue. In the standing sequences, these are the hill pose, wherby the feet are kept together; the triangle pose, in which the feet are kept apart by about three to four feet; and finally one-legged balancing poses. In the seated sequences, they are the asymmetrical sequence; the symmetrical posterior stretch sequence; the meditative poses, built around the *vajrasana* (thunderbolt) pose; and the classical lotus pose. Then are inverted poses, such as the headstand and the handstand, all in one sequence. The lying-down poses form another important sequence, as does the sequence consisting of supine (lying face-up) poses. Additionally, there are special sequences like the sun salutation. All these sequences make yoga practice a very rich experience, and yoga a consummate art.

Asana practice is done for health and to reduce the rajas, or the tendency in us to engage in uncoordinated physical activity and distractions of the mind. The vinyasa krama is given full treatment in Ramaswami's book, *The Complete Book of Vinyasa Yoga*. This chapter is organized to proceed from general practice to specific sequences and it roughly follows the order of that book, so we suggest you refer to the book for further guidance.

❧ BREATH IN ASANA ❧

(See the introduction to *The Complete Book of Vinyasa Yoga*)

DAVID: What is the difference between doing asana with long, slow breathing and doing asana with a hold after inhale and exhale? Is one a preparation for the other? Is the real goal to do asana with long, slow, smooth breathing?

For example, what is the difference between doing asana with the breath ratio 5:5:5:5 (inhale for 5 seconds, hold for 5 seconds, exhale for 5 seconds, hold for 5 seconds . . .) and doing asana with the ratio 10:0:10:0 (inhale for 10 seconds, do not hold, exhale for 10 seconds, do not hold . . .)?

63

RAMASWAMI: Doing asanas with long inhalation and exhalation is peculiar to vinyasa krama. You do all the movements either with inhalation or exhalation. Very rarely do you hold the breath in vinyasa krama. There are a few exceptions, such as *suryanamaskara* (sun salutation). Here, you want to use the mantras in between vinyasas, and it is good to hold the breath while chanting or reciting the mantra. Sometimes one may stay in a vinyasa holding the breath for a short while. And in vinyasa krama, the number of times you do a movement is limited to, say, three times or so.

On the other hand, sitting in a classic asana, one does inhalation, holding, exhalation, and holding out in *pranayama* (yogic breath control), without movements as in vinyasa krama. Thus the vinyasa krama method of doing asanas, in which long inhalations and exhalations are used, is actually a very good preparation for pranayama (or *kumbhaka*). In systems where breathing is not used in asana practice, that is, where people breathe freely without control, sometimes hurriedly under strain (which is the normal contemporary practice, except for the teachings of Sri. T. Krishnamacharya), it is a lot more difficult to learn pranayama, and, as a result, many schools seldom teach it.

So the 5:5:5:5 or 10:0:10:0 ratio, with respect to pranayama, usually done in a classical seated pose such as *padmasana* (lotus pose) or *siddhasana* (accomplished pose). According to Patanjali, two of the parameters of pranayama are: *dirga* (long) and *sukshma* (fine or nice or smooth) breathing. So, from this point of view, it is clear that longer time in each aspect of breathing is definitely recommended. I feel that the minimum duration is 5:5:5:5.

When equal time is used for all the aspects, especially inhalation and exhalation, it is called *samavritti pranayama*. The popular ratio 5:20:10:5 is called *vishamavritti* (unequal duration). This, naturally, requires more control. Depending upon the requirements of the student, the ratio can be changed. For instance, for youngsters, a longer holding in period will be beneficial, as it helps to expand the chest and improve concentration. For older people, longer exhalation will be useful, for it helps them to relax. So, depending upon the requirements, the ratio will have to be modified. The texts give only sample ratios and are not exhaustive.

DAVID: In general, should we make inhale and exhale equal (in length) when moving into and out of forward bends and twists, but when we stay in a forward bend or twist, make inhale short and exhale long? Can we say the reverse about backbends?

RAMASWAMI: Mostly in forward bends, it is easy to extend your exhalation, and so the *abhyasi* (one who practices) can take advantage of the forward-bend position to lengthen and smooth the exhalation. And in forward bend, deep or full inhalation is more difficult, again because of the position: the stomach cannot freely expand to accommodate fuller breathing and hence we would do a shorter inhalation.

Can we say the similar things about inhalation, will the converse be true? Bending back is a different cup of tea. While it is natural and beneficial to do fuller inhalation while bending back, for some backbends done while in a prone position, such as the cobra or locust pose, the inhalation could restrict the backbend due to the pressure on the expanding abdomen. So, many people, primarily the obese and/or tense, are advised to do backbends on exhalation (*langhana kriya*). We may therefore say that, although inhalation is the breathing of choice in backbends, there are compelling reasons for some practitioners to use exhalation for these movements.

If we really want to work on our inhalation it may be best to do it while practicing pranayama in a cozy seated pose such as vajrasana or padmasana.

DAVID: In vinyasa krama, we usually make the inhale and the exhale equal in length. But are there times when we alter this? For example, if students need to relax, would we encourage them to practice with emphasis on exhale, making their exhale longer than their inhale? And, conversely, if a student needs to build confidence, open his/her chest, increase his/her inhale, etc., would we encourage practice with emphasis on inhale?

Or, should we ignore all this and simply recommend long, slow breathing?

RAMASWAMI: While exhalation can be extended in forward bends in vinyasa krama, and one may practice to lengthen the exhalation while doing a series of vinyasas, it may not be easy or productive to work on inhalation in vinyasa krama. It is best to work on inhalation in a seated posture while preparing for or doing pranayama.

DAVID: Do we ever think about an asana practice in terms of the number of breaths taken? What number of breaths is a good, average practice? Within a practice, for example, how many breaths of backbending should we do?

RAMASWAMI: While doing asanas in the vinyasa method, you can stay in a few vinyasas, such as *parsva bhangi* (side poses) or *utkatasana* (hip squat), or some backbends such as *makarasana* (crocodile pose), for a few breaths, say, three to six breaths. But in more involved poses, such as *paschimatanasana* (posterior stretch pose) or *sarvangasana* (shoulder stand), one may stay for a long time, say, ten to fifteen minutes. If the breath rate is good, say, 2 to 4 per minute, you can decide to stay for a certain number of breaths, say, 30 to 60 breaths. The idea should be to stay longer with the minimum number of breaths as possible.

DAVID: What does the word *pranasthana* mean?

RAMASWAMI: Empirically, *pranasthana* refers to the locus, the point or location within the chest, from which inhalation appears to start and exhalation appears to end. It is the center of breathing. *Prana* means "breath." *Pra* is "manifest" and *ana* is "to breathe." And *sthana* means "the place or location."

DAVID: In asana, the mind follows the breath. Does this again mean to focus on the pranasthana?

RAMASWAMI: Yes, that is what one should attempt to do. But many people will find it more convenient to follow the breath in the throat; because the *ujjayi* sound (yogic breathing with constriction in throat) and the rubbing sensation in the throat will help them to focus on the breath more easily at the throat.

DAVID: I've been told that it's safe to do any asana movement on exhale, even backbends. But the reverse is not true. We cannot do every movement on inhale. Why is this?

RAMASWAMI: The general rule is to use inhalation during backbends and in stretches involving raising arms and extending legs. Naturally, inhalation cannot be used in movements involving contraction of the body, such as forward bends or twists, because in contraction movements we would like the internal muscles also to contract rather than expand, so these have to be done without inhalation, which would impede the contraction. As I mentioned earlier, exhalation in backbends is resorted to in cases of people who are tight, who may have problems like hypertension, and who are generally obese. Expansion movements should logically be done with inhalation, but in the cases I have just mentioned it may be better to do them on exhalation. Exhalation tends to relax the muscles.

DAVID: Sometimes, in order to work on the breath, I'll exhale first, then move into *uttanasana* (forward bend) on hold after exhale. The same procedure applies to *trikonasana* (twist). Also, as a way of working on the breath, sometimes I'll break the inhale or exhale into two or more steps (*krama*). Are these techniques not used in vinyasa krama?

67

RAMASWAMI: Yes, sometimes it may be easier to move when holding the breath. But as a rule, the movement should accompany breathing in or out. Of course there are specific circumstances when you may have to hold the breath in or out during a brisk movement; e.g., the jumping movements in suryanamaskara or some such movements in the Ashtanga yoga vinyasa krama. If you are comfortable breaking the breath to complete one movement, you may do so. However, basically one should find a rhythm or speed of movement that is slow. The pace should be such that there is no strain in the breath necessitating breaking the breath into two parts in the course of one movement. In the initial stages of practice, 5 seconds for each movement will be ideal. The breath will not be too strained and the movement not too hurried. Furthermore, during the practice, if you find that the breath has quickened and you tend to compensate by breaking the movement to have another breath, maybe it is time to take a short rest period.

DAVID: Occasionally, in a vinyasa krama sequence, we move on hold after exhale. For example, in the *paschimatanasana* (posterior stretch pose) sequence (see chapter 3 of *The Complete Book of Vinyasa Yoga*) we may lie down, exhale completely, and then, suspending the breath, move into paschimatanasana. Is the purpose of this to strengthen and deepen the exhale? Might we not do the same with uttanasana? Exhale completely after raising our arms and then, on hold after exhale, move into uttanasana?

RAMASWAMI: Basically, some of the movements are done easily, at least in the initial stages, if you hold the breath. When one tries to sit up from the lying-down position, one normally holds the breath and comes up with a bit of effort. So for many beginners, it will be easier if they hold the breath to come to paschimatanasana from the *supta asana* (lying-on-back pose) position. But after some practice, it should be possible for the practitioner to anchor the heels nicely and come up while smoothly exhaling. So the holding of the breath is an initial concession. It could apply to other situations also.

The use of breath holding is useful in some therapeutic applications. The mini sequence: *tadasana* (hill pose)—utkatasana-uttanasana-utkatasana-uttanasana—(repeat a few times)—tadasana can be attempted by holding the breath after exhalation for the duration of the sequence. After three or four such movements, you may rest in tadasana and collect your breath. This is a langhana kriya (exhalation) sequence and is helpful in correcting marginal obesity.

I would say anything other than long inhalation/exhalation in vinyasa krama would have to be attempted only in specific cases requiring some special effect, usually for therapy.

DAVID: If we want to do utkatasana as a separate asana, to stay and lengthen *bahya kumbhaka* (hold after exhale), when would we do it? After the tadasana sequence?

RAMASWAMI: The better or easier posture to extend your bahya kumbhaka would be apanasana (pelvic floor pose).

DAVID: Why do you say apanasana is best for working on bahya kumbhaka? Is it because here the body is contracted, which is conducive to long exhale?

RAMASWAMI: I mentioned apanasana in the context of using

utkatasana for developing the bahya kumbhaka. With a better, stabler base, it is easier to do bahya kumbhaka in apanasana than utkatasana, in which it may be more difficult to stay.

DAVID: In asana, when we do a vinyasa sequence that requires jumping, do we jump on hold after exhale or inhale? For instance, in the sun salutation, we jump on hold after inhale from utkatasana to catarunga, and again from downward-facing dog to utkatasana, on hold after inhale. But, I've also done sun salutations where we jump from uttanasana to chatarunga on hold after exhale. And, in trikonasana, we jump the legs apart on hold after exhale. Or, are these just guidelines and really we can do either?

RAMASWAMI: This can be answered better by understanding the reasoning behind the synchronization of breath and movement in vinyasa krama. All expansion movements are usually done while inhaling and all contraction while exhaling. When you raise the arms, you do it with inhalation. When you stretch the legs or bend back, it usually is done during inhalation. Likewise when you bend the knees and draw the legs toward your body, as in utkatasana or apanasana, it has to be during exhalation. Dropping your arms down or twisting the body or bending the body will be done with exhalation. When you do an expansive movement, such as raising the arms, if you also inhale, not only the muscles of the limbs stretch but also the muscles inside the chest expand with the inhalation. Thus, there is both an internal and external stretching taking place. This is *anuloma* (with the grain movement). On the other hand, if you do it without proper breathing, the full advantage of coordinated stretching is not obtained. Similarly, when you contract the body, as in bending forward, if you exhale it becomes easier to contract the internal muscles as you contract the external muscles.

Now, jumping is not a common occurrence in yoga practice. Since jumping is a swift movement, you cannot synchronize it

69

with the breath as we do in slow vinyasa movements. So we hold the breath while jumping. Here, also, the reasoning will be to keep the internal muscles stretched as you stretch the external muscles. So when you jump from utkatasana to *chaturanga-dandasana* (four-legged staff pose), since there is an extension of the body and also the chest, it is logical to do it with internal breath holding. The same will be the case if you jump from uttanasana to chaturanga-dandasana. In the case of trikonasana, since only the legs are involved and not the chest, it is okay to jump after exhalation.

There is one more point to note. as discussed, people who are older or who are obese find it difficult to inhale and do some of the extension and backbending movements simultaneously. Applying the same logic, some may be advised to do the jumping from utkatasana to chaturanga-dandasana while holding the breath out after exhalation. But it is better not to ask older or obese people to jump as kids do.

BRAHMANA AND LANGHANA KRIYA

DAVID: In the version of the *Yoga Makaranda* that I have, Krishnamacharya, in writing about asanas, states, "Those who are overweight should follow langhana kriya (activity of reduction) and those who are underweight should follow brahmana kriya (activity of expansion)...In brhmana kriya, the breath is held in after inhalation, for some time, before exhalation. This is known as antah kumbhaka. In langhana kriya, the breath is held after exhalation, for some time, before allowing air in. This is known as bahya kumbhaka." Is this different from the way you were taught?

RAMASWAMI: The Sanskrit word *brahmana* means "to grow, to expand," whereas *langhana* means "to reduce, to diminish back to its cause." So exhalation is considered langhana and inhalation is considered brahmana kriya. Actually, inhalation is expansion of the chest, and holding the breath keeps the chest expanded, so both will be brahmana kriya, whereas langhana kriya is the opposite of it.

❧ BANDHAS IN ASANA ❧

DAVID: What is the purpose of bandhas in asana? Is it just to practice and perfect them for pranayama? Or, do they have a function in asana practice?

RAMASWAMI: Among other things, *bandhas* (locks), especially *mula bandha* (rectal lock), help to pull up the pelvic floor and also to pull the pelvis off the hip joint. *Uddiyana bandha* (abdominal lock) helps stretch the lumbar spine and *jalandhara bandha* (chin lock) helps to stretch the whole spine, especially the thoracic spine.

Of course there are several other advantages, but purely looking from the point of view of asanas, the bandhas help to perfect the posture.

DAVID: Why do we keep the chin down, in jalandhara bandha, in most of the tadasana sequence? (See chapter 1 of *The Complete Book of Vinyasa Yoga.*) In your first book you say that jalandhara bandha helps with our balance. I think it also stretches the cervical vertebrae. In some cases, it may protect the heart. In YR I, 71, 72 a more esoteric reason is suggested: that jalandhara bandha blocks the flow of *amrtam* (nectar).

RAMASWAMI: You may also consider this point. In vinyasa krama, since the breathing is controlled to synchronize with the movements, it is necessary to control the breath at some point in the respiratory track. The hands are used in *nadi sodhana* (cleansing the pathways), but since the arms also move in most of the vinyasas, the best way to control the breath will be in the throat, by partially closing the glottis, producing the ujjayi effect. The head-down position better achieves controlling the throat breathing.

Hatha Yoga Pradipika and several other yoga texts also talk about the prevention of the amrita being consumed by the gastric fire, and jalandhara bandha prevents it. The term *jalandhara bandha* implies the sealing of the flow or leakage of amrita.

DAVID: Why is the chin not kept down in a twist or lateral bend? Is this because of balance?

RAMASWAMI: Basically, in twisting, the whole spine should come in to play. That means that the cervical spine also should move, in tandem with the rest of the spine. Consequently, the head also turns with the turning of the cervical spine and neck.

DAVID: There are two versions of *urdhva-mukha swanasana* (upward-facing dog pose), one with the chin down and one with the head back. What is the difference? Which one is preferred?

RAMASWAMI: My teacher used to ask us to do the pose with the chin lock. The chin lock helps to stretch the spine. This is also a pose where you are required to stay for a while and hence the preferred position of the head is to maintain jalandhar bandha. You may also add the head back movement as an additional variation. In fact it will be good to maintain jalandhara bandha in the three poses of the sequence, consisting of *adho-mukha swanasana* (downward-facing dog pose), chaturanga-dandasana, and urdhva-mukha swanasana. You may extend this sequence to include *halasana* (plough pose), which is an excellent pose for jalandhara bandha (see *The Complete Book of Vinyasa Yoga*, page 242).

DAVID: Can we do mula and uddiyana bandhas in a twist?

RAMASWAMI: Yes, my teacher used to ask us to do mula bandha and uddiyana bandha in jathara parivritti (belly twist), a good twist pose. One is encouraged to do the mula bandha and uddiyana bandha is such postures as *Matsyendrasana* (Matsyendra's pose). Since the bandhas and some of the seated twists, such as Matsyendrasana, are said to help in the arousal of *kundalini* (energy as coiled serpent), it may be correct to introduce the two bandhas in twists, as they work in tandem.

❧ PSYCHOLOGICAL BENEFITS ❧ OF ASANAS

DAVID: Patanjali's YS II, 48 states, *"tatah dvandva anabhighatah"* (the practice of asana makes us unaffected by the opposites, like heat and cold). Is this also true of the mental opposites, like praise and criticism? How does this happen?

There are those who have practiced asanas for many years but are still stung by criticism and become enraged. Is this because they are not yet strong in yama niyama, especially Isvarapranidhana?

Is the idea that practice of asana reduces rajas and that, as Aranya uggests, pain is a form of restlessness?

RAMASWAMI: Adi Sankara mentions that when rajas impinges on satwa, pain results. So if one can reduce the power of uncontrolled rajas, by practicing asanas slowly as in Vinyasa krama, then the rajas will come down, hopefully giving way for satwa. The pairs of opposites, or *dwanda*, include both physical and mental pairs. It is said that such a yogi who has rajas under control is not easily affected by the pairs of opposites, like heat and cold, at the physical level, or praise and ridicule at the mental level. Actually, both the pairs are felt by the mind, the chitta. To be affected by the pairs of opposites indicates a state of intolerance, which is a manifestation of rajas, according to Samkhyas and several authors. Actually, to be affected by dwanda is an indication of predominance of rajas. Asanas should help to reduce that. But if the yogi continues to live in conditions that enhance rajas, such as rajasic food or nonyogic association, then the effect of asana practice in reducing rajas could be affected.

DAVID: You point out that Adi Sankara says: When rajas impinges on satwa, pain results. Where does Sankara say this? In one of his commentaries?

RAMASWAMI: Yes, in his *Vivarana* (explanatory work) to Vyasa's commentary on the *Yoga Sutras of Patanjali*.

DAVID: Will a practice with emphasis on inhale increase courage, confidence, strength (*virya*)?

RAMASWAMI: Inhalation and, more important, breath-holding after inhalation, are said to be energizing. Actually, the pranayama mantra, which contains Gayatri, an energizing mantra, is used while doing samantraka pranayama. That is why we have the 1:4:2 ratio suggested. But then it is best done in a seated pose as part of a regular pranayama practice.

DAVID: Do the balancing postures, the one-legged (*ekapada*) sequence (*The Complete Book of Vinyasa Yoga*, chapter 4) and the hand balances (*The Complete Book of Vinyasa Yoga*, pages 172–75), really have anything to do with our psychological balance? How so?

RAMASWAMI: I think the balancing poses help to develop a more acute sense of balance. Since we know that. in a state of panic or distress, we tend to lose physical balance and scramble to sit down, we may say that learning to improve the sense of physical balance will have a positive effect on the mental stability as well.

REDUCING RAJAS AND TAMAS

DAVID: We have been saying that the practice of asana reduces rajas and pranayama reduces tamas. But, in his commentary on

HYP I, 17, Brahmananda says that asana removes the heaviness in the body that is caused by tamas. Should we say that pranayama removes the tamas in the mind and asana removes the tamas in the body? But then doesn't YS I, 31, "*duhkha daurmanasya angame-jayatva* . . ." (mental pain, depression, trembling of limbs . . .), equate the two? If we reduce the tamas in the mind, we will have reduced it in the body and vice versa?

75

RAMASWAMI: What you say is correct. When we say that asana removes rajas, it means that the primary function of asanas is to remove the rajas. The same passage of *Brahmananda* you refer to clearly indicates that asanas remove rajas (*asanena rajo hanti*). This is found in one of the minor Upanishads also. Further in the *Yoga Sutras*, the benefit of asana practice is said to be the endurance of the pairs of opposites. Affliction of dvanda referred to here is the manifestation of intolerance, which is rajasic. And Patanjali in the *Yoga Sutras*, explaining the benefits of pranayama, indicates that pranayama helps to remove the covering (*avarana*) of the chitta. Avarana refers to tamas, as seen from *Samkhya Karika* (text on Samkhya philosophy) as well.

It is to be construed that though we talk of the gunas as separate characteristics, most of the time one guna is predominant while the others support it. So in this case, purely from practical point of view, and also based on experience, Swatmarama and Brah-mananda say that removal of tamas also takes place by the practice of asanas. In the system of vinyasa krama, since we use both breathing and movements simultaneously, one can say with assurance that both tamas and rajas can be reduced by asana practice.

ON PRACTICE

DAVID: Is it best to have sarvangasana (shoulder stand) come toward the end of our practice? For example, if we are doing both the paschimatanasana sequence and the supta asana sequence (*The Complete Book of Vinyasa Yoga*, chapter 5) including shoulder stand, then should we do (a) the paschimatanasana sequence, followed by supta asana including shoulder stand; or (b) the supta asana sequence including shoulder stand, followed by paschimatanasana? Does the order matter?

RAMASWAMI: Adaptation of the sequence will vary from person to person and also by the individual's requirement at a particular time. The sequencing I have suggested in my book and programs is for learning.

DAVID: In Vinyasa Krama, could we do the supta asana sequence and shoulder stand (with counterpose) followed by the vajrasana sequence (*The Complete Book of Vinyasa Yoga*, chapter 9)?

RAMASWAMI: Yes, if you have the correct reasons for that.

DAVID: You say that, in vinyasa krama, we can reverse the normal order and do the vajrasana sequence after supta asana and shoulder stand, if we do it for the correct reasons. Would give an example of reasoning that would lead to this conclusion?

RAMASWAMI: For instance, if you would like to use vajrasana for pranayama and *dhyana* (meditation), which you may plan to do after practice of asanas.

DAVID: In general, what is the proper order of sequences in a practice? May we freely alternate standing, seated, lying, and so on?

RAMASWAMI: There is scope for changing the order of sequences, but it cannot be done randomly. The practitioner should reason out why he/she is doing a particular sequence or why he/she wants to change a particular routine.

DAVID: Why is it better to determine our course of asana practice before we begin? What's wrong with jumping around, doing whatever asana feels right to do next? Do we lose focus, concentration, direction? Are we, in some sense, being led by the senses, when we simply do whatever "feels right"? Would this be taking us in a direction away from kaivalya?

RAMASWAMI: Satwa is order and tamas is disorder. So in all activities, it is good to bring some order and hence it is suggested that we should determine beforehand what we want to do during our yoga practice, like having an agenda for a meeting.

77

In fact, in all religious activities in India, it always starts with *sankalpa*, a clear-cut determination about what one is going to do. Even when chanting Gayatri, there is a sankalpa—one would say that one would do so many times: 32, 64, 108, or 1,008 of Gayatri mantra repetitions, or *japa*. Almost all religious, meditation, and pranayama activities have this sankalpa.

Even the commentator to *Hatha Yoga Pradipika* refers to the sankalpa before starting the practice of yoga. One should ponder a little before starting one's practice and have a definite agenda of practice. A random practice is not conducive to orderly thought process. And subsequent practices, such as *dhyana* (meditation), all require a disciplined mind. It can start with a determination of a definite course for practice.

DAVID: There are so many vinyasas of sarvangasana and sirsasana—we can't do them all every day (can we?). How do we decide which ones to do?

RAMASWAMI: It is necessary to program every day's practice so that one will be able to practice all the vinyasas over a period of time. It may be a good idea to practice some asanas with vinyasas for a while, and stay in important poses. It is just a question of proper planning and using the time judiciously.

DAVID: It is quite common for a student to come to me and request a half-hour practice. What do you recommend in such a case?

RAMASWAMI: Fifteen to twenty minutes of several vinyasas—movements with breathing—will be good. One can possibly do about 50 to 60 movements during that time. It can be followed by some pranayama and shanmukhi mudra (sealing the six senses).

Another day, it could be some asanas such as sarvangasana or paschimatanasana, where one can stay for about 3 to 5 minutes.

78

DAVID: If I am working my way through one of the vinyasa krama sequences and my mind becomes distracted and I forget to do one of the asanas in the sequence, should I go back and do that asana (out of order) when I remember it? Or just forget about it for that day and continue through the rest of the sequence?

RAMASWAMI: You may very well continue with the practice rather than breaking the sequence to return to the vinyasa inadvertently missed.

Staying in Poses

DAVID: In vinyasa krama, we stay in most of the asanas for only a brief time. But there are three—inversions, paschimatanasana, and *maha mudra* (the great seal)—that we stay in for a longer period. Why is this? I can understand that the inversions are thought to have great benefits, but why are paschimatanasana and maha mudra thought to give greater benefit than other asanas?

RAMASWAMI: In vinyasa practice, several of the vinyasas are facilitators of the main pose, so they are done for a few times. But the purpose of vinyasa krama is to make one fit to do and stay in an important posture for a long period of time. Vajrasana, the lotus pose, and other meditative poses require that you stay in the pose for a long period of time for doing pranayama or meditation. Asanas that are important are mentioned in several yoga texts, such as *Hatha Yoga Pradipika*.

In some cases, the guru would recommend that a particular student should stay in a pose for a long time because of the therapeutic effects of the pose, as is the case with the inversions. In fact, Swatmarama (author of *Hatha Yoga Pradipika*) specifies that one should virtually live in paschimatanasana. Maha mudra is not considered an asana, though it has to be considered in the asymmetrical seated posture sequence. In HYP, maha mudra is considered the best of all mudras. My guru used to say that one should stay in maha mudra for a long time, as it helps to direct the vital energy through appropriate nadis. However, vinyasa krama does not specify the duration one has to be in a posture, or even in a vinyasa.

DAVID: With such asanas as utkatasana in the tadasana sequence, and maha mudra in the asymmetrical seated sequence, it's better not to stay in the asana in the sequence, but to stay in them separately. Why is this? For balance? Harmony? But we do stay in paschimatanasana for some time in the paschimatanasana sequence.

RAMASWAMI: It is difficult to have cut-and-dried rules for specific situations. In the paschimatanasana sequence, paschimatanasana is the main asana or the centerpiece, and all the preliminary movements will have helped to achieve the posture, which may not be the case if you get to paschimatanasa without the preliminary movements. Maha mudra is a comparatively easy pose. And utkatasana is a pose in which you can stay for a while, but not as long as one would stay in paschimatanasana.

DAVID: Should the three asanas we stay in for some time— inversion, paschimatanasana, and maha mudra—be done every day?

RAMASWAMI: Yes. These poses are very effective ones, so it will be advisable to practice them every day. Serious students of yoga, who would like to use yoga not merely for maintaining health and peace of mind but want to work toward the higher goals mentioned in the Sastras (scriptures), should commit themselves to yoga virtually as a life goal and lifelong practice. Long hours of practice and deep study are necessary.

Rotation of Hip Joint

80   **DAVID:** In the padmasana sequence (see chapter 10 of *The Complete Book of Vinyasa Yoga*), when we twist and bend forward toward one knee (figure 2-1), for the return we first rotate to the center and then come up. Is this for a more complete rotation? In *upavishta konasana* (seated-angle pose) (figure 2-2) and in trikonasana we have similar movements where we first twist and then bend forward. Here, as well, we could make the return movement by first rotating to the center and then coming up. Is this done sometimes?

RAMASWAMI: Yes, we can do that. But, since this rotation movement for the hip is more effective in the *urdhva konasana* (raised triangle pose) (see figure 2-3) in sarvangasana, we would try to make use of the free position of the hip joints for rotation.

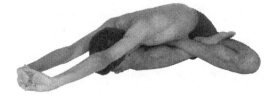

FIGURE 2-1

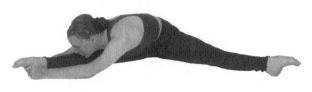

FIGURE 2-2

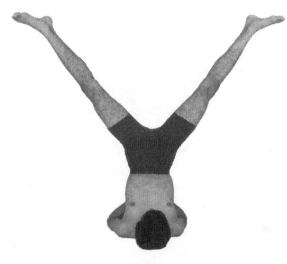

81

FIGURE 2-3

Overcoming Difficulties in Attaining Poses

DAVID: When we find tightness in an asana, how do we proceed?

RAMASWAMI: The only known way to overcome tightness in a posture is to follow a vinyasa krama sequence. The difficult pose may be preceded by several preparatory movements with proper breathing. Doing many movements, going into a posture and doing variations in a posture, will all work on several muscles that we may not be able to consciously work on. And, once one gets into the pose, one may try to do a few movements or vinyasas with proper breathing. This would be helpful.

DAVID: Are there any suggestions for overcoming fear in asana, for instance, in some inversions such as headstand, handstand, or *pincha mayurasana* (stretched-feathers peacock pose)?

RAMASWAMI: According to *Hatha Yoga Pradipika*, the general advice for success in asana practice consists of six factors. They are:

꙰ zeal (*utsaha*)

꙰ perseverance (*sahasa*)

꙰ courage (*dharya*)

꙰ knowledge (*tatwagnana*)

꙰ clarity (*nischaya*)

꙰ a certain aloofness (*janasanga parityaga*)

82

The six undesirable traits for the yogi are:

꙰ gluttony (*atyahara*)

꙰ exertion (*prayasa*)

꙰ talkativeness (*prajalpa*)

꙰ certain debilitating vows such as continuous fasting (*niyamagraha*)

꙰ socializing or partying (*janasangha*)

꙰ vacillation (*laulya*)

The commentator also refers to excessive physical activity, such as carrying heavy loads or weight-lifting or practicing too many sun salutations. These, too, should be avoided.

I think a slow, step-by-step approach like Vinyasa krama affords an excellent way of overcoming fear. Learning to do sarvangasana well would be a nice preparation for headstand. Here again, one can learn to practice headstand in steps: supporting oneself against a wall or transferring the weight to the head with the help of the teacher. Relaxed shoulders and a nice smooth curve of the backbone will help achieve the stability so essential in headstand. Staying in akunchanasana (contraction pose) and getting a feel for the head-down position are good first steps. I think most people can do headstand if the technique is properly understood.

Prishtanjali

DAVID: When we do a forward bend with the hands in *prishtanjali* (the back salute), on return we bend back. Why not with other *hasta* (hand) vinyasas (variations)? We can also arch and bend back with the hands in other positions, such as interlocked overhead, can't we?

RAMASWAMI: When the hands are in prishtanjali, the shoulders are already opened up and hence the torso is already slightly opened up. It is easy to do this back bending and will be a comfortable way to open the chest.

It is not exactly the case with the arms overhead. One has to deliberately push back the arms to bend back.

❧ ASANAS IN DIFFERENT SEQUENCES ❧

DAVID: In each asana we can forward bend, twist, and backbend. So which do we use, and for what purpose? That is, what is the difference between forward bend in tadasana and forward bend while lying down? What is the difference between twisting while standing and twisting while lying down?

RAMASWAMI: Most important poses lend themselves to the movements you mention. But obviously different groups of muscles will be exercised differently in different poses even for the same movements of the torso. Furthermore, as you could see, these movements could be more difficult in tadasana than in the lying-down position to a less healthy person. Again, backbends are easier done in some seated poses or even while standing than while lying down. A forward bend while standing could help stretch the legs more than in a seated forward bend, where the legs are on the floor and cannot be pushed back as in the standing position. Obviously, while the bends and twists refer to the torso, the position of the lower extremities and the pelvis will have different effects.

David: There was one practice we did together which went like this: some of the trikonasana series, a few supine asanas, a few prone asanas including dhanurasana, then *baddha konasana* (bent-knees straight-angle pose) with forward bending, *kapalabhati* (rapid abdominal breathing), pranayama, and shanmukhi mudra.

I was surprised to see baddha konasana in the practice. I thought it was part of the paschimatanasana sequence, yet here it is isolated. Is baddha konasana being used, in this case, as *pratikriya* (counterpose)?

Ramaswami: I think we may have done maha mudra followed by baddha konasana because it is logical to do baddha konasana after maha mudra. Baddha konasana can also be part of the paschimatanasana series, for it is a logical extension of upavishta konasana and *samakonasana* (straight-angle pose).

In vinyasa krama, some of the asanas come in different sequences. Adho-mukha swanasana can be a part of the Sun salutation series and also part of *Vasishtasana* (Vasishta's pose) series or for that matter dandasana (staff pose). Likewise urdhva padmasana (lifted-up lotus pose) can be part of padmasana sequence and also sarvangasana sequence.

✿ MAIN POSE ✾

David: In some of the vinyasa krama sequences there is a main pose, and the vinyasas help prepare us for it. Thus, as discussed, the vinyasas in the paschimatanasana sequence clearly help prepare us to stay in paschimatanasana for a long time. But, in other sequences, there does not appear to be a main pose. For instance, is there a main pose in the trikonasana sequence (*The Complete Book of Vinyasa Yoga*, chapter 7)? Or in the vajrasana sequence? Are these sequences helping to prepare us to stay in some pose?

RAMASWAMI: In some sequences, we may identify one pose in the main sequence, but in some others, such as trikonasana, there can be a few more, each subsequence having an important pose. In trikonasana sequence, we will have trikonasana, uttita parsva konasana (side stretch triangle pose), and virabhadrasana (warrior pose) as important poses. In the tadasana sequence, the last posture, tadasana, in which you raise the heels, is the important one. But, in between, we pass through several other main poses, such as uttanasana, utkatasana, and others, each having their own subsequences but still blending with the flow of the main sequence.

85

❧ TADASANA SEQUENCE ❧

DAVID: In the tadasana sequence (see chapter 1 of *The Complete Book of Vinyasa Yoga*), when we raise our arms from the front (second movement), we do not interlock the fingers and turn the palms up. Is this because doing so would rotate the arms and change the effect of the movement? Is it correct that when we raise the arms from the front, the effect of the movement is on a different (lower) part of the back?

RAMASWAMI: Yes, in this movement, if you attempt to interlock fingers, you will have interrupted the flow of the movement toward the end. Thus, whenever you want to interlock fingers after raising the arms, it will have to be done laterally. As you say, it stretches the back toward the end of the movement. It helps to stretch the front portion (purva bhaga) of the body very well.

DAVID: If we are doing parshva uttanasana, the forward bend to the side where we first twist and then bend, where does this come in the tadasana sequence? After uttanasana?

RAMASWAMI: After uttanasana.

DAVID: If we are practicing *pasasana* (noose pose), should it come after utkatasana and before the final tadasana in the sequence?

RAMASWAMI: Yes, pasasana involves both the squat and the twist, so it is better to do it after doing utkatasana. In the final tadasana, the main joints involved are the ankles, which we can attend to after we have worked on the hip joints (which is facilitated by utkatasana).

DAVID: If we are doing a partial version of *tiryang-mukha uttanasana* (standing complete back stretch pose), for instance, just bending back and touching a wall behind, where does this come in the tadasana sequence? At the end?

RAMASWAMI: We can do this after we complete the forward bend and as the last of the uttanasana sequence, before we proceed to do ardha and full utkatasana.

DAVID: On page 221 of *Yoga for the Three Stages of Life*, you mention an asana, sankatasana (figure 2-4). What is this?

RAMASWAMI: It is another name for *ardha-utkatasana* (half-squat or chair pose).

DAVID: When I move into ardha-utkatasana, in order to bring the thighs parallel to the ground, the chest moves toward the legs. Is it more important to have the thighs parallel to the ground, or to have the back further back and more upright?

RAMASWAMI: Parallel thighs and feet on the floor are more important.

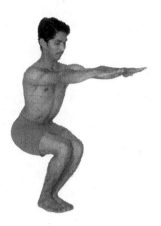

Figure 2-4

❧ SAVASANA ❧

DAVID: HYP I, 32 states that *savasana* (corpse pose) induces repose of mind. Did Krishnamacharya ever use savasana for this purpose? Have you?

RAMASWAMI: I found that my guru would ask us to take to savasana (figure 2-5) for rest and recovering breath after some strenuous exercises that would sometimes quicken the breathing. It usually would be for a brief period.

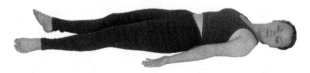

Figure 2-5

❧ ASYMMETRICAL SEATED SEQUENCE ❧

DAVID: In the asymmetrical seated aequence (see *The Complete Book of Vinyasa Yoga*, chapter 2), maha mudra is done without a counterpose. Or, is janu sirsasana considered a counterpose for maha mudra?

88

RAMASWAMI: Maha mudra is included as part of the asymmetrical sequence, in one of the progression of the asanas, even though it is not strictly an asana. Because of the position of the bent leg, any backward bending (which could be a counterpose) will be awkward, as there is no proper anchor for the bent leg. It's a different story when the bent leg is in half lotus or Marichyasana (Marichi's pose) or tiryang-mukha (backward facing) poses. Then there is a proper anchor, and a counterpose can be done.

Janu sirsasana (head-on-knee pose) is not a counterpose for maha mudra. Furthermore, in maha mudra, there is little forward bending to really warrant a backbend as a counterpose.

DAVID: In HYP I, 27, it is stated that Matsyendrasana prevents the loss of amrita. It is easy to imagine how sirsasana might do this, as it is an inversion. But how does this happen with a twist? Is this why Matsyendrasana (figure 2-6) is held in such high regard?

RAMASWAMI: Celibacy is considered an important ingredient of spiritual life in many religions and communities. Some of the poses, such as Matsyendrasana and Brahmacharya, go hand in hand. That is, if you practice poses like these you may be able to maintain celibacy, and conversely if you maintain celibacy you can master these poses. Matsyendrasana, by working powerfully on the pelvic floor and the base of the spine, could help maintain celibacy by controlling the nadis that discharge vital energy, according to yogis. We have seen that gastric fire wastes amrita when it falls down due to gravity. Such asanas as sirsasana arrest this downward movement, and consumption of amrita is prevented. This is the ideation.

Seminal discharge, likewise, is considered to be loss of amrita. Hence yogis of the Hatha school and Kundalini school suggest the reversal of the downward movement and discharge of the vital energy, and the forcing of it upward. They found this was not possible due to the blockage of the *sushumna* (the spinal pathway) by kundalini. As long as kundalini blocks the sushumna, the vital energy goes down and out. So they worked toward clearing the passage of the sushumna by the arousal of kundalini. Once that is done, the vital energy controlled by *apana* (a physiological force in lower region of the body) is made to unite with *prana* (the life force), and both move up and merge with the Siva principle in the *sahasrara* (a chakra) in the head. Of course, this is an ideation. So people who follow this procedure are also known as urdhva retas, or urdhva retaska (those who take the vital energy [*retas* = semen] upward).

So Matsyendrasana is considered to be good for preventing the loss of cool ambrosial nectar.

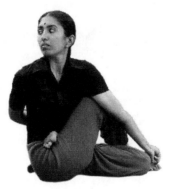

Figure 2-6

DAVID: Is there a reason why we always start asymmetrical asanas on the right side? Or, doesn't it matter?

RAMASWAMI: It is customary to do the movement on the right side and then the other side, not only in seated asymmetrical postures but also in other sequences such as the one-legged standing sequence, or parsva bhangi (side poses), and others. Maybe it is because most of us are right-handed. Sometimes, when I used to do the posture starting from the left side, my teacher would ask me to start from right side.

90

✑ PASCHIMATANASANA SEQUENCE ✑

DAVID: Do you feel paschimatanasana (see *The Complete Book of Vinyasa Yoga*, pages 75–77) should be done every day?

RAMASWAMI: If you find the time, it should be given preference in practice. Many find it an easier forward stretch than uttanasana, because of the better stability of the pose.

DAVID: You say that many find paschimatanasana an easier forward bend than uttanasana because of the stability of the pose. I can see that, but, if stability standing is not a problem, wouldn't uttanasana be easier because the hips are allowed to move back, whereas in paschimatanasana the hips are blocked by the floor?

RAMASWAMI: Precisely. The point is that, even though several poses look alike, the effects could be substantially different. That is one reason why vinyasa krama is important because no two vinyasas give the same result.

To take some extreme examples, the body can be kept straight in tadasana (figure 2-7), *danda samarpana* (prostrating) (figure 2-8), supta asana (figure 2-9), or sirasasana (figure 2-10). You could see that all have different effects. Tadasana may help align the chakras, sirasasana will help the repositioning of internal organs, supta asana or its savasana variant will help one to relax, and danda samarpana brings out the emotion of surrender.

Other similar-looking asana groups could be paschimatanasana (figure 2-11), *urdhva-mukha paschimatanasana* (upward-facing posterior stretch pose) (figure 2-12), urdhva paschimatanasana (figure 2-13), and uttanasana (figure 2-14). Another group will be utkatasana (figure 2-15), apanasana (figure 2-16), *akunchanasana* (contraction pose) (figure 2-17) in sirasasana, and forward bend in vajrasana (figure 2-18). The effects on each asana in each group could be substantially different even though they look alike.

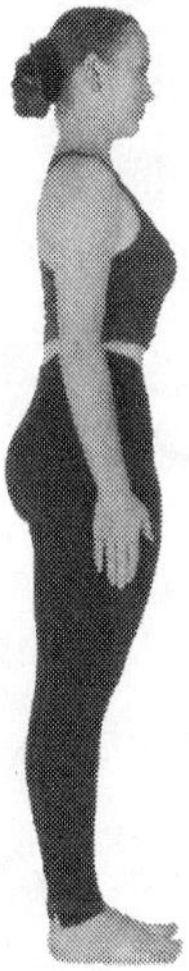

91

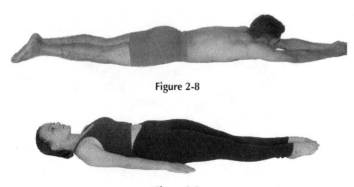

Figure 2-7

Figure 2-8

Figure 2-9

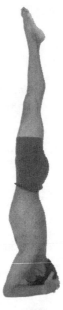

Figure 2-10

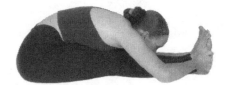

Figure 2-11

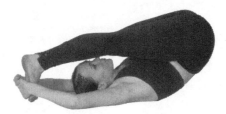

Figure 2-12

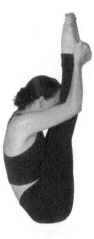
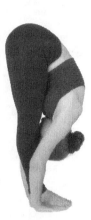

Figure 2-13   Figure 2-14

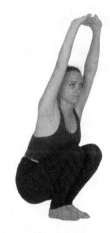

Figure 2-15

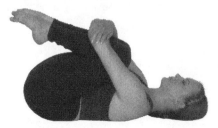

Figure 2-16

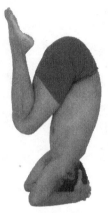

Figure 2-17

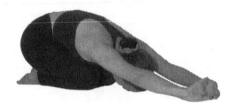

Figure 2-18

DAVID: Is it best to use some of the asymmetrical seated postures sequence (e.g., ardha-padma paschimatanasana) as prep for paschimatanasana? Or, can we simply begin the paschimatanasana sequence directly?

RAMASWAMI: I think, when you start learning asana practice, it will be good to prepare the body well with asymmetrical seated sequences before venturing into the symmetrical sequence of paschimatanasana. The asymmetrical sequence helps to correct the body on either side, lest in the symmetrical sequence there may be disproportionate stretch on either side.

DAVID: Is baddha konasana (figure 2-19) also considered a counterpose for samakonasana (figure 2-20)?

RAMASWAMI: The progression of subgroups in the paschi-matana sequence will be the legs together position as in paschi-matanasana, then the upavishta konasana subroutine, ending with samakonasana. In all these, the legs are kept stretched. So it may be a good idea to do baddha konasana as a counterpose, to give some relief to the hamstrings.

DAVID: This is a question on the various hasta vinyasas in paschimatanasana, With some, such as when arms are extended to the sides at shoulder height, we can begin from the supta posi-tion and move into paschimatanasana on exhale. But with others, such as prstanjali, we would have to start from dandasana and move to paschimatanasana. Is this correct? With some we would begin from supta, with others from dandasana?

RAMASWAMI: Normally the movement into paschima-tanasana from supta asana is done with arms extended overhead, mainly to get some leverage and momentum to do the forward bend, especially for beginners or at the start of the paschi-matanasana practice. The ususal starting point for paschi-matanasana is dandasana. Thereafter, the movements are done from dandasana. Such special vinyasa sequences as halasana, paschimatansana, and uttana mayurasana are generally helpful toward stretching the body very well.

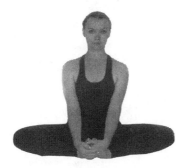

Figure 2-19

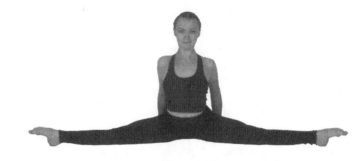

Figure 2-20

DAVID: In catushpada-pitam (table pose) (figure 2-21), is the idea to bring the heels as close to the butt as we can?

RAMASWAMI: Yes, in which case you will be able to raise the hip quite fully. Furthermore, it will help to anchor the feet well as you raise the trunk. I think the correct position of the feet is such that the legs are straight when you complete the pose.

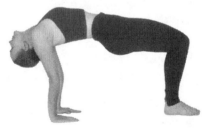

Figure 2-21

❦ EKAPADA SEQUENCE ❦

DAVID: Why, in ekapada (one-foot) postures, do we bring the palms together overhead instead of interlocking the fingers?

RAMASWAMI: You can do these poses with interlocked fingers. But the one-legged standing poses, or balancing poses, are also known to be used by *tapasvins*—those doing penance. One well-known pose of this kind is Bhagiratasana (figure 2-22). Bhagirata was a king and he wanted to get the waters of Ganges to flow down the plains from the Himalayas, so that the river would flow over the ashes of his forefathers, who were condemned and cursed due to their act of extreme disrespect to a pious sage. Only the pure waters of Ganga could give them salvation. He did penance to please Lord Shiva to let Ganga flow down to the plains. Ganga was considered the consort of Shiva and was perched on the matted hairs of Shiva.

97

So in these poses the hands are held together in anjali mudra (palms together). Normally, we keep the folded hands in front of our heart, and most householders are supposed to keep the anjali mudra in this fashion. But tapasvins, recluses, sanyasins, and maybe some renunciate yogis, keep the arms up and the hands in anjali mudra, as requiring more effort. Some call it *urdhwanjali* (when we keep the hands behind our back in anjali, we call it *prishtanjali*). So keeping the hands high and together in anjali mudra, while in balancing poses, is more than a mere technicality.

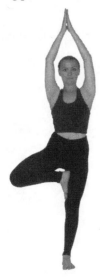

Figure 2-22

DAVID: When we do *ekapadangushtasana* (balancing on one leg and holding the big toe with the fingers) do we keep the head down? For some time, I thought it helped with the balance to look forward and stare at a spot on the wall. But now, I do the asana with head down and stare at a spot on the floor. This seems to work well and I think this is what you recommend in *The Complete Book of Vinyasa Yoga.*

RAMASWAMI: Yes. Keeping the head down while keeping the back straight will help maintain good balance. It is all the more useful in one-legged poses such as Bhagiratasana, and ekapadangushtasana (figure 2-23). My teacher always used to stand erect but usually keep the head down. The way he used to walk is something one should emulate: His back would be straight, even in his advanced age, but his head would be kept down. I think it is a good practice, especially for the elders, because you are likely to maintain a better balance and the chances of falling down are less. (I hope I will remember this, as I am getting older.)

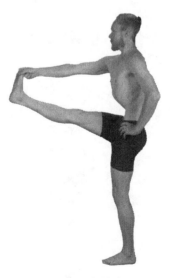

Figure 2-23

In India, with its uneven footpaths, roads, and terrain, it is a good practice to have your eyes on the road rather than looking around. Gotama, the author of *Nyaya Sutras* (a Vedic philosophical text on law and logical thinking), was also known as Akshapada, the one with his eyes on his feet, indicating that he had his head down. Certain sects in India committed to Ahimsa as the great vow will walk with their heads down, lest they trample upon ants, insects, or worms while walking, and thus break the vow.

DAVID: Is *garudasana* (eagle) part of the ekapada sequence? In garudasana, do we try and stand up straighter with each inhale? Or, do we keep the knee bent but try and straighten the back?

RAMASWAMI: I had not thought about it. I think straightening the back will be helpful.

SUPTA ASANA SEQUENCE

DAVID: In apanasana (see *The Complete Book of Vinyasa Yoga*, chapter 5), when I bring both knees to the chest and wrap my arms around, then, if I keep the lower spine and tailbone on the floor, my head and chest are off the floor. Is it more important to have the tailbone and spine on the floor, or to have the head and upper back on the floor?

RAMASWAMI: It is important to keep the head on the floor for apanasana (see figure 2-24), and one may move the head and neck in pavanamuktanasana (wind-release pose), the different head position vinyasas. (see figures 2-25, 2-26, 2-27).

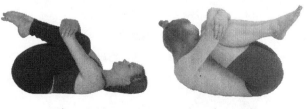

Figure 2-24   Figure 2-25

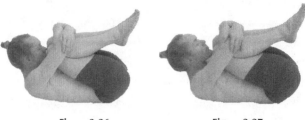

Figure 2-26   **Figure 2-27**

DAVID: When we're opening the legs in *supta konasana* (lying supine with the legs spread) (figure 2-3, page 81) or when we're lowering the leg to one side in *supta padangusthasana* (holding toes with the fingers in the lying-down position), are we free to do so on either exhale or inhale, as there is neither contraction nor expansion of the trunk?

RAMASWAMI: Yes you can, but it is better or safer to use exhalation in all these movements, even if the chest is not directly involved. When in doubt, or have a choice, use exhalation or langhana kriya.

DAVID: Is the asana called *uttana-padasana* (raised-leg pose) part of the vinyasa krama system? Should we be very cautious about the neck in trying this?

RAMASWAMI: Uttana-padasana (see figure 2-28) is a complete spine-bending exercise, *without support*. The crown and the buttock bones should be properly anchored and there is no half measure in this pose. With the arms and legs stretched up, the whole upper body should be absolutely relaxed to be able to do this pose without a mishap. It is a pose that one should start learning early in life, and it may be rather difficult to start after middle age. It is part of the supta asana vinyasas or variations in lying-down position. Done independently, the counterpose for this pose will be Apanasana. The neck and upper body should be

well conditioned by doing several of the hasta vinyasas mentioned in *The Complete Book of Vinyasa Yoga*, pages 4–13.

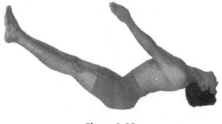

Figure 2-28

❀ SARVANGASANA ❀

DAVID: How do we know if someone's neck is ready for the person to try sarvangasana (shoulder stand) (figure 2-29)?

RAMASWAMI: One of the reasons that many people refrain
from doing sarvangasana is that they are afraid that they may
harm the neck due to the overextension. Furthermore, when we
are tense, it is the neck that becomes stiff. Doing asana with a
"spastic" neck is very unpleasant, and the ill effects linger for a
long time. I have found that good exercise to the arms, shoulders,
neck, and the torso can be obtained by the hasta vinyasas in a posture like, say, tadasana. Please refer to *The Complete Book of Vinyasa
Yoga*, chapter 1. I also find that if a person can stay in shanmukhi
mudra (closing of all the ports) for about five minutes in a yogic
pose such as lotus or thunderbolt, without feeling any stiffness in
the neck or shoulders, he/she will be able to do sarvangasana
comfortably. Some long exhalations (*rechaka*) before sarvangasana also could be helpful. Any time one feels tight and anxious,
it is better to avoid sarvangasana. Also, in such conditions as
spondylosis, the pose should be avoided.

So, to practice sarvangasana one must be very relaxed.

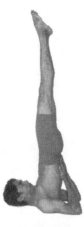

Figure 2-29

DAVID: If sarvangasana is part of our daily practice, are we free to choose any vinyasas of shoulderstand we please? Or, should we, for instance, do akunchanasana every day?

RAMASWAMI: We must understand the purpose of vinyasa krama. When you practice asanas in this method, the whole body gets the workout. If you look at the whole gamut of asanas and vinyasas, you will find that, by assuming different poses and moving within the parameters of a posture through the vinyasas, the yogis have developed a system so that the whole body is taken care of, including the internal organs. So, one has to practice vinyasas as much as possible to be able to stay in a pose. And later on, from continued practice, one can stay for a long time, even forgetting one's own body at the time of internal practices (*antaranga sadhana*) such as meditation or samadhi. Random methods of exercising the body, such as doing a few asanas without vinyasas, will never get the perfection in a posture. People shun lotus pose, thunderbolt, shoulderstand, and so on, mainly because they cannot stay in such poses for a long time. Without achieving comfort in these poses, further yoga progress becomes difficult. The answer to "Why do vinyasa krama?" can be summarized as follows:

1. Without the movements in classical poses you cannot master those poses.
2. Without the mastery of these poses, the higher practices of yoga cannot be attempted.

DAVID: Can we use salabhasana (figure 2-30) (locust pose) and/or dhanurasana (figure 2-31) as a *pratikriya* (counterpose) for sarvangasana? Or, is it best to always use makarasana (crocodile pose) (figure 2-32) and bhujangasana (cobra pose) (figure 2-33)? Why are these considered pratikriya for sarvangasana? It seems they work mostly on the back; do they also work on the neck?

RAMASWAMI: Salabhasana and dhanurasana require you to raise the lower extremities apart from raising the chest and bending back the neck. However, we need not require the leg movement in the counterpose to sarvangasana. We have to relieve the strain the neck due to the exaggerated bending of the neck in sarvangasana. In makarasana and bhujangasana, the leg movements are not there, though in some variations we can use the lifting of the legs. But in simple bhujangasana and makarasana, only the neck is bent back. Furthermore, the arms or palms are on the ground supporting and helping to control the movement, which is different from the situation in salabhasana and dhanurasana. Both salabhasana and dhanurasana are more difficult poses, and we should choose a very simple pose for a counterpose. The counterposes, as a rule, should be simple, effective and targeted. Bhujangasana and especially makrasana will be ideal, better than dhanurasana or Matsyasana (kingfish pose) (figure 2-34), as some suggest, for a counterpose to sarvangasana.

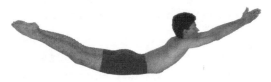

Figure 2-30

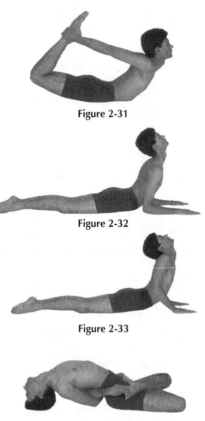

Figure 2-31

Figure 2-32

Figure 2-33

Figure 2-34

DAVID: When I'm in sarvangasana, if I extend myself fully, straightening the upper back and stretching the legs completely, then my breath is shorter. If I relax a bit, my breath is longer. Which is preferable?

RAMASWAMI: If the stretch starts right from the neck, goes all along the spine, and then extends to the lower extremities, the breath may not get shorter. The shoulder also should be relaxed.

DAVID: What is *parsva pindasana* (side-fetus pose)?

RAMASWAMI: *Pindasana* (fetus pose) done on the side (figure 2-35).

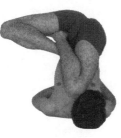

Figure 2-35

❧ THE INVERTED POSTURE SEQUENCE ❧

DAVID: How long should we stay in headstand? How long in sarvangasana? Are there guidelines? Should we just follow the breath, as usual? Come down when the breath grows short, and rest? Can we go back up as often as we like?

RAMASWAMI: I can give some general ideas, based on my experience with my teacher. It is good to stay at least for five minutes in headstand. Because of the nature of the pose, the body takes a little longer to adjust, start relaxing, and enable gravity to work on the internal organs and also several of the skeletal muscles.

In headstand, the breathing rate also is very important. Shortness of breath indicates straining, and is not good. If the breathing gets longer and smoother as you stay in the posture, it will be more effective. Correct postural alignment also is necessary to stay in the posture. If all these things are taken into consideration, anywhere between 15 and 30 minutes will be good. Some people decide to stay for a definite number of breaths and try to keep the breath as long as comfortable. A breathing rate of about four per minute will be good; two per minute will be somewhat of a Siddhi (accomplishment). One can introduce the mula and uddiyana bandhas to enhance the effectiveness of the pose for the internal organs. After some time staying in the pose, one may attempt some variations, such as akunchanasana, urdhva konasana, urdhva padmasana, and so on.

Several years back, when I was very young, I saw a yogi who I heard would stay in headstand for three hours a day. He was maintaining silence, so I could not get any details. But his face had a dark bluish hue, indicating some blood stagnation. So, I think about half an hour at a time will be long enough. But if one wants to practice for that long, the neck should be supple and without any problems. Also, the eyes should be normal; and the blood pressure.

106

In the initial stages, going up and down a few times will help to get to know the correct position of the head, so it is relaxed and has proper alignment. While going up and coming down, it will be good to maintain correct balance throughout, without tightening the neck and shoulder muscles. Making use of the relaxed spine by rounding it will be a good method to maintain and adjust the pose.

DAVID: Why are the inversions not in *Hatha Yoga Pradipika*?

RAMASWAMI: My understanding is that they were so intricate that it is necessary to learn them only directly from a teacher and not from books or hearsay. HYP does mention such inversions as viparita karanai (upside-down exercise), and says that they should be learned from a guru.

DAVID: How long should the pratikriya of sarvangasana be? Should this equal to the amount of time spent in headstand?

RAMASWAMI: Sarvangasana is used as a counterpose to retain the benefits of headstand a little longer. One theory is that, in headstand, the amrita is made to stay in the head rather than drip down and be consumed by the *jatharagni* (gastric fire), as happens while we stand or sit up. To retain the nectar in the head and to help amrita to spread in the head, sarvangasana, another topsy-turvy pose, is used for a short period as a counterpose. I am used to doing sarvangasana as a counterpose for a short period, say, for about 5 minutes, after a headstand practice of anywhere between 15 to 30 minutes.

DAVID: Is akunchanasana done in handstand? If so, do we then go up into handstand from akunchanasana just as we do in headstand and shoulderstand?

RAMASWAMI: In shoulder stand and headstand, the head/ head and shoulders are anchored, so it becomes easy to round the spine and achieve akunchanasana. But, in handstand, the head is floating, and hence it is difficult to round the spine and achieve good akunchanasana (figure 2-36).

Handstand, and standing on the forearms, is ideally suited to do many backbending exercises such as pincha mayurasana or *vrischikasana* (scorpion pose) (figure 2-37). Since the head and neck are free to move in these poses, much better backbending becomes possible in handstands, than in head- and shoulderstands.

107

One may be able to akunchanasana in handstand, but it may be awkward.

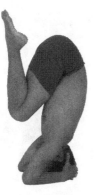

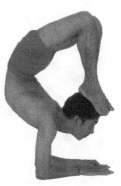

Figure 2-36   Figure 2-37

TWIST IN TRIKONASANA

DAVID: Once we have some mastery of twist in trikonasana, can we then go into the twist in one movement? Or, is it best to continue doing the twist in three parts?

RAMASWAMI: It is better to do the trikonasana twist in three parts even after one becomes very competent (figures 2-38, 2-39, and 2-40). The three-part movement works on different groups of muscles, and it is safer and more beneficial than doing the asana all in one movement. The one-part approach is a physical train-ing approach, like the drills done in schools.

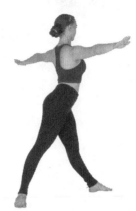

Figure 2-38

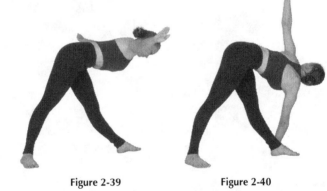

Figure 2-39   **Figure 2-40**

✿ VAJRASANA SEQUENCE ✿

DAVID: After doing *virasana* (hero's pose) in the vajrasana sequence (see chapter 9 of *The Complete Book of Vinyasa Yoga*), would it make sense to then do Marichyasana with one leg in tiryang mukha, and kraunchasana (heron pose) with one leg in virasana position, even though these vinyasas are usually found in the asymmetrical seated sequence?

RAMASWAMI: Since we consider vajrasana and virasana to be symmetrical poses, the asymmetrical variations are not normally introduced. But I have seen my teacher ask us to go up to the kneeling position in vajrasana (figure 2-41), stretch one leg forward (figure 2-42), and slide/sit down to tiryang mukha (figure 2-43) It is considered another method of getting to tiryang mukha pose, or it can be considered a lead sequence. So it is okay to try these variations. The Marichyasana is one step away.

109

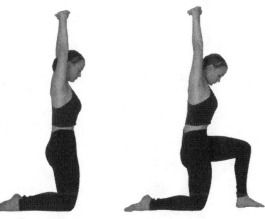

Figure 2-41   Figure 2-42

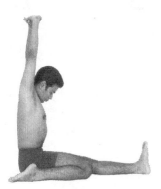

Figure 2-43

DAVID: Forward bends in vajrasana can be done from two starting positions, seated on the heels or up on the knees. We usually do the forward bends from the seated-on-the-heels position, but some movements, such as bending the elbows, we start from up on the knees. Is one starting position preferable to the other? Why do we use one or the other?

RAMASWAMI: Forward bends in vajrasana are done from the seated-on-the-heels position. The elbow-bending movement is sequenced as follows: Start from the seated vajrasana position. Inhale, raise the arms as you raise the trunk and stand on your knees (see figure 2-44). Then, as you exhale, return to the seated position while bending the elbows (see figure 2-45).

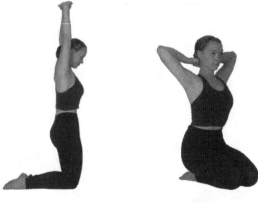

Figure 2-44   Figure 2-45

DAVID: In vajrasana, we do all the forward bends from the seated-on-the-heels position. Why then, for the bending of the elbows, do we come up to standing on our knee? We could just as well extend the arms and bend the elbows from the seated-on-the-heels position.

RAMASWAMI: We can do the arm-bending movement seated. But in the one under reference, we are also raising the hips. These two movements complement each other, the arm-bending movement and the lowering of the trunk from the kneeling position.

DAVID: Why do we cross the legs for *simhasana* (lion pose)? Why not just do it in vajrasana?

RAMASWAMI: This is a posture in which the legs are crossed and the heels are placed on either side of the generative organ. Maybe the sage who developed the asana found that his simhasana resembled the way the lion sat (see figure 2-46).

111

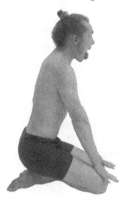

Figure 2-46

❧ VISESHA SEQUENCES ❧

The following questions and answers refer to chapter 11 of *The Complete Book of Vinyasa Yoga*.

DAVID: In your answer on the chin lock in urdhva-mukha swanasana (figure 2-47), you say this is a pose you are required to stay in for a while. When and how is this done? Is this one of the visesha sequences? Is the same true for adho-mukha swanasana (figure 2-48) and chaturanga -dandasana (figure 2-49); that is, do we also stay in these for some time?

RAMASWAMI: As mentioned earlier, these three poses form a nice sequence and, with halasana (figure 2-50), form an extended visesha vinyasa sequence. One method of practice is to stay in each one of the three (or four poses) for several breaths, maintaining jalandhara bandha.

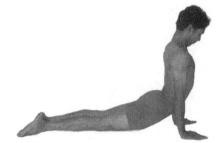

Figure 2-47

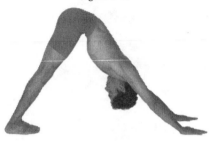

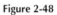

Figure 2-48

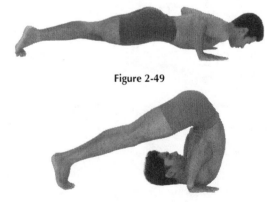

Figure 2-49

Figure 2-50

DAVID: How often do we do the visesha sequences? Occasionally, for variety? Or, more systematically?

RAMASWAMI: Sequences such as suryanamaskara or *dingnamaskara* (salutations to the directions) can be done regularly or on specific occasions. One may also select some sequences if one thinks that the particular sequence will meet certain specific requirements. It may be a good idea to include some special sequence almost daily.

DAVID: In the vinyasa krama method, which sequence does Vasisthasana (Vasishta's pose) belong in? Or, is Vasisthasana the beginning of its own sequence?

RAMASWAMI: Vasishtasana (figure 2-51) can be done independently starting from dandasana. One *visesha* (special/unique) vinyasa sequence involves doing Vasishtasana from the hub pose, *adho-muka swanasana* (downward-facing dog pose): go to Vasishtasana with left hand up, proceed to do purvatanasana (anterior stretch pose), and then go to Vasisthasana on the other side (right hand up). The appropriate breathing will have to be followed. You end the sequence by coming down to adho-mukha swanasana. You may do the same movements in the reverse order to come to the starting point.

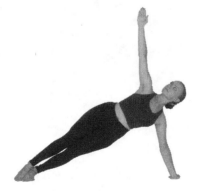

Figure 2-51

❧ JATARAPARAVRITTI AND KONASANAS ❧

DAVID: YR I, 52 says that there are three variations of jataraparavritti and also three variations of baddha konasana and other konasanas (stomach twist and angle poses). Are these just different vinyasas? What are they?

RAMASWAMI: *Jataraparivritti* means twisting of the abdomen (*parivritti* = complete activation). So some poses where this effect is prominent have been designated as jataraparivritti. The simplest of them is shown in my book *The Complete Book of Vinyasa Yoga*, page 106. Two more jataraparivritti are shown here (figures 2-52 and 2-53).

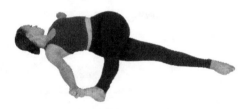

Figure 2-52

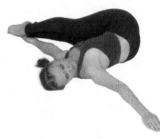

Figure 2-53

Likewise, baddha konasana and konasana. *Konasana* is to keep the legs in a triangle formation, spread about 45 degrees. The following page numbers refer to CBVY. Examples of different konasanas include urdhva konasana (page 128 and 166), upavishta konasana (pages 81 and 82), parsva konasana (page 150), and trikonasana (page 147). Baddha konasana is also considered a variation of konasana. My teacher dictated to me a verse from *Yoga Rahasya*. It says that the five konasanas are useful during pregnancy. For more details you may refer to page 216 of *Yoga for the Three Stages of Life*.

115

❧ MAYURASANA ❧

DAVID: In YY III, 15–16, *mayurasana* (peacock pose) is given as one of the important asanas. Is this because of how beneficial it is for digestion? Also, for this and several other asanas, the text uses the phrase, "destroys all impurities." How are we to take this? It seems like a rather extreme statement.

RAMASWAMI: Mayurasana (figure 2-54) is given considerable importance by several yogis. Even many *puranas* (epics) and other nonyoga texts refer to this posture. It would appear that it was one of the prominent postures known for a long time.

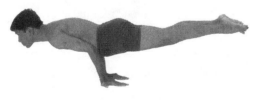

Figure 2-54

According to Yagnavalkya, the lower abdomen, the pelvic region, known as *kandasthana*, is a breeding ground for many diseases. And mayurasana, by its very nature, imparts considerable pressure on this region. So, even if it may appear rather sweeping to say that it destroys all impurities, this statement is not entirely off the mark. When I was a young boy, I heard it said by many elders that mayurasana would help improve digestion and also help in cases of diabetes. But it is a very difficult pose to master.

✏ VYASA'S ASANAS ✏

DAVID: In Vyasa's commentary on YS II, 46, he lists a number of asanas. Some of these are familiar to me (if they have their usual meanings); others are strange. What is sopasraya? Is paryanka what we refer to as paryankasana? Is krauncha-nisadana the same as what we call krauncasana? What is hasti-nisadana?

RAMASWAMI: *Sopasraya* is *sa* + *upa* + *asraya*. As *asraya* or *upasraya* means "support" or "substratum," we can take this word to mean broadly "with support." Many experts indicate that *sopasraya* can mean the use of a platform or wooden plank with a blanket or deer or tiger skin spread on it, for use in asana practice. Modern yogis may be inclined to include as well the many intricate props under the term *sopasraya*.

Nisadana means "resemblance." So *krauncha nishadana* would mean a posture that resembles a *krauncha* (heron).

Hasti means "elephant," so *hasti nishadana* can be called the "elephantlike pose." *Paryanka* is "couch," and here paryankasana would mean a couch pose (figure 2-55).

So it is with *ushtra nishadana* (camel) (figures 2-56, 2-57)

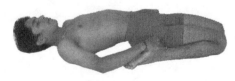

Figure 2-55

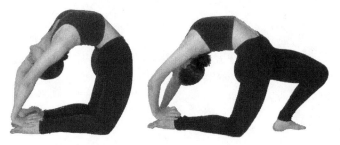

Figure 2-56   Figure 2-57

117

✿ MAHA MUDRA ✿

DAVID: Maha mudra is one of the essential postures, one we stay in for some time. It comes naturally in the asymmetrical seated sequence, but we may not want to stay in it for some time at that point in the sequence. When can maha mudra be done, if we want to stay in it? At the end of the sequence? Can we do it after the paschimatanasana sequence? Or at the end of our practice, and stay in it then for some time?

RAMASWAMI: If you go by *Hatha Yoga Pradipika*, maha mudra (figure 2-58) can be done after pranayama (kumbhaka) practice. But then, when you practice yoga for a long time, and since you use breath and the bandhas in vinyasa krama practice, you may be able to do maha mudra at any time. Maha mudra can be used to practice the bandhas after pranayama also. I think it is best to practice long duration maha mudra at the end of asana session. Some people do not do maha mudra in the asymmetrical sequence but do only janu sirsasana in that sequence—and do maha mudra separately as a mudra and not as an asana.

DAVID: What is the minimum preparation (*purvanga*) for maha mudra?

RAMASWAMI: A good workout of the asymmetrical sequence will be a good preparation for maha mudra. Also kapalbhati (rapid abdominal breathing) and *recaka* (long exhalation) will also be helpful.

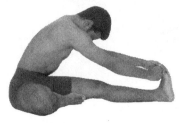

Figure 2-58

DAVID: Can we do maha mudra after pranayama?

RAMASWAMI: If you go by *Hatha Yoga Pradipika*, since maha mudra is a mudra, it can be done after pranayama. As I have mentioned earlier, vinyasa krama practice combines asana, breathing, and some of the mudras.

DAVID: Why is baddha konasana considered a counterpose for maha mudra?

RAMASWAMI: Normally it is good to do baddha konasana after maha mudra and janu sirsasana, because it harmonizes with them. The hip joints open out nicely in baddha konasana after they are stretched individually in maha mudra. And since in maha mudra one stays for a long time, it will be a good relief to do baddha konasana as a follow-up procedure.

DAVID: You suggest practicing long duration maha mudra at the end of an asana session. So, for example, would this be a typical practice: tadasana sequence, lying-down sequence including shoulder stand, counterpose for shoulderstand, rest, maha mudra for some time, then pranayama?

RAMASWAMI: Yes, it is acceptable.

DAVID: You also mention doing maha mudra separately, as a mudra and not as an asana. Is the idea that mudras are done after pranayama, but before meditation? What is the difference between doing it as a mudra and doing it as an asana?

RAMASWAMI: I think I have explained it already. If you want to work on maha mudra and stay for a long time, you can do it at the end of the session even after pranayama, because you will be concentrating on the bandhas. The pranayama, especially the long exhalation, will improve the quality of the mula and uddiyana bandhas. If you do maha mudra as part of the asymmetrical seated sequence, you may stay for just a few breaths.

119

❧ FURTHER Q&AS ON PRACTICE ❧

Utpluti

DAVID: Is utpluti (lifting) always done on hold after exhale?

RAMASWAMI: I think it is more comfortable and safer to do utpluti while holding the breath after exhalation.

DAVID: Why do you think it's safer to do utpluti on hold after exhale? Is there some danger in lifting the body on inhale?

RAMASWAMI: It is easier after exhalation, because one tends to be less tight after exhalation. Normally, breath-holding after inhalation pushes down the diaphragm, makes the the chest full. I think it is easier to do utpluti while breath-holding after exhale.

Jump-Throughs

DAVID: In the Yoga Makaranda, Krishnamacharya has given vinyasas to go from samasthiti to many asanas, such as paschimatanasana, ardha padma paschimatanasana (half-lotus with backbend), and tiryang-mukha ekapada-pascima-uttanasana (backward-facing one-foot posterior stretch pose). These vinyasas all involve jump-throughs. Were these primarily meant for children? In the vinyasa krama sequences I've learned from you, once we begin a sequence we proceed to the next asana without returning to samasthiti each time.

RAMASWAMI: *Yoga Makaranda* is not a complete book on vinyasa krama. There, my guru had included several, but a limited number, of the difficult and spectacular poses and movements, such as the jump-throughs. If on a particular day you want to practice tiryang-mukha uttanasana (standing complete backbend), the approach will be to start from samasthiti and go through the various steps of vinyasa krama. On another day, if you are going to practice paschimatanasana and on yet another day Marichyasana, you have to start from samasthiti, and go through the steps. So, in that book, he dealt with each of the seated poses separately and has given the procedure. The book does not say anything to preclude one from doing several seated poses in one sitting, in which case you would get to dandasana from samasthiti and complete whatever asanas/vinyasas you would like to do while seated. Furthermore, the book does not include all the vinyasas in any one particular pose like tiryang-mukha or ardha padma. There are several more vinyasas he would teach routinely in each of these seated positions, which are not found in the book.

Tiryang

DAVID: Sometimes I see the word *tiryang* (backward) spelled *triyang*. Which is the correct spelling?

RAMASWAMI: *Tiyak* or *Tiryang* in a compound word (as in tiryang-mukha) is right.

120

Eyes

DAVID: Are there any asanas or movements suggested for the eyes?

RAMASWAMI: Shanmukhi mudra (figure 2-59) would be very relaxing to the eyes. Trying to do *bahis trataka* (external gazing) by looking into a *deepa* (lamp or flame) with the eyes kept open until they water, is a practice my teacher used to recommend. And then keeping the image of the deepa after closing the eyes is internal (antah-trataka, or internal gazing). Some schools suggest having two flames on either side in front and moving the eyes from one to another.

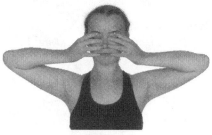

Figure 2-59

Maha Vedha

DAVID: In describing *maha vedha* in HYP III, 27, Svatmarama seems to talk about a kind of bouncing on the ground. Am I picturing this right?

RAMASWAMI: Slowly, gingerly.

Adjustments

DAVID: When Krishnamacharya taught, would he demonstrate asanas for students? Would he make adjustments when the student was in an asana? Mohan told me that one day Krishnamacharya demonstrated sixty-six vinyasas of sirsasana for him.

RAMASWAMI: Yes, he used to make adjustments when necessary,

when absolutely necessary. When he was teaching for our family, he would help my father with some movements, but more extensively for my brother who was slightly physically challenged. In the initial stages of my learning, he used to stand behind me and support my low back and legs while teaching sarvangasana and sirsasana.

Toward the latter part of his life, he used to do very few demonstrations, and many were done by his students—once my sister demonstrated ushtrasana and sarvangasana to some visiting yogis under my guru's instructions.

Yes, sirsasana, along with sarvangasana and padmasana, lends itself to several variations. I have included scores of variations in my book *The Complete Book of Vinyasa Yoga*, especially for sirsasana.

DAVID: You say Krishnamacharya would only make adjustments when absolutely necessary. Why do you think this was? Did he feel perhaps that it was best if the student learned for him/herself? Did he feel that yoga itself was the best teacher and that doing your practice, following the precepts of *sthira* (stability) and *sukha* (comfort), would lead one to the right posture? Or, was it something else?

RAMASWAMI: I think it is a good policy to give directions orally first, then if necessary demonstrate and finally help the student. I thought my guru wanted to involve the student/patient as much as possible for his/her good.

Dangers

DAVID: In the commentary to HYP I, 14, Brahmananda warns us that in Hatha yoga, a mistake may end in death or insanity. Can this be? I once did hear, secondhand, of an American student who had a breakdown after attempting to gain mastery of kechari mudra.

RAMASWAMI: One has to give sufficient weight to these warnings. Some of the Hatha yoga practices, such as vajroli or amaroli mudra, do not find favor with orthodox people in India because, except for the very strong willed, these could lead the young yogi astray. Some Tantric practices, when done improperly, can affect the mind. People compare practicing yoga to walking on a razor's edge. But the advantages of correct, sincere practice are numerous. Sometime back, I heard a neurosurgeon talk about a case he came across. It would appear that a middle-aged man learned headstand from a teacher and was practicing it regularly. He had such faith in his master and his headstand that he never felt it necessary to have a medical checkup, even when he started feeling somewhat unwell. He later on was found to have pronounced hypertension. One day he stood in headstand for about fifteen minutes, came down from his posture, immediately had a stroke, and died.

I also know of cases where people without prior yoga practice go to yogis for therapy and come away with a false sense of security: that with yoga everything will be fine. But should a fifty-year-old novice jump through his/her hands? Is the same set of limited asanas appropriate for all the people all the time? Appropriate practice is the key to success in yoga. That was what my guru would emphasize.

Age of Vinyasa Krama

DAVID: Is the vinyasa krama method old? Even ancient? I wonder because there were no others besides Krishnamacharya teaching it.

RAMASWAMI: According to my guru, the vinyasa krama is old. The word *vinyasa*, itself, is old and used in several arts, such as music and painting.

Since I had only one teacher, I am not able to know if others also taught it.

Anyway, I think it is wonderful to learn, practice, teach, and savor vinyasa yoga.

3

On Pranayama

INTRODUCTION

PRANAYAMA IS ONE of the best innovations of yogis. *Pranayama* means "lengthening of the breath" and also "control of the breath." Since the simple process of breathing is under both voluntary and involuntary control, the yogis realized that by making the breathing process more and more under voluntary control they could control the physiological and mental processes. A variety of practices that help control each aspect of breathing—exhalation, inhalation, and holding and releasing the breath—were worked out and diligently practiced. The yogis invented myriad variations of pranayama practice by changing the place of control, time duration for the different phases of breathing, and/or the number of pranayama cycles in each sitting.

Pranayama reduces the *tamo* guna (physical and mental inertia) and, along with asana practice, helps clear the system of the rajas and tamas. The result is that you become very satwic—the ideal condition for the rewarding process of meditation.

Pranayama also has several physical and physiological benefits.

It expands the chest, improves the vital capacity, and helps slowly overcome several respiratory ailments such as bronchial asthma, shortness of breath, and irregular breathing. Along with the bandhas and mudras, it improves blood circulation to and into the heart. Pranayama practice is referred to even in the Vedas, the ancient scriptures. Among old-timers in India, it is a traditional practice to make an offering of food to the Lord, and to the five pranas (life forces). Pranayama is also used to prepare for meditation by using appropriate mantras—the mantras may be from the Vedas or specific personal deities. No meditation, according to traditional yoga, can be done without a prior good stint of pranayama.

125

Pranayama requires considerable attention. First, you should choose a proper seated posture so that you may stay steady in the pose without discomfort or disturbance for the long time needed to practice pranayama and then meditation.

More information on pranayama practice can be found in the yoga books of Srivatsa Ramaswami, *The Complete Book of Vinyasa Yoga* and *Yoga for the Three Stages of Life*.

BREATH AND PRANA

DAVID: YY VI, 35–38 says that retaining the prana within the body is called *pranayama*. Is prana (or some of it) normally outside the body? Is it dispersed and needs to be gathered?

RAMASWAMI: The meaning of *pranayama* is "restraining the breath": *prana* (the breath, or life force) + *ayama* (to lengthen, or restrain). Pranayama is usually associated with restraining the breath inside, which is called *antah kumbhaka*. This is what Yagnyavalkya has indicated here. Even the *Hatha Yoga Pradipika* uses the word *kumbhaka* (restraining/holding the breath) as the heading of the second chapter on pranayama.

DAVID: In YY VI, 39–49, Yajnavalkya speaks of the benefits of focusing the prana at various places in the body. First of all, how is this done? Is the idea that by focusing the mind at a particular place, the prana will flow to that place? (Here again, we have the idea of the prana moving.) Second, these benefits must be of great use in yoga chikitsa (therapy). For example, it is mentioned that by focusing on the navel, all diseases are removed, by focusing on the big toes lightness is acquired, and so on. So, the practice of *bhavana* (ideation) in pranayama would seem to be of great practical benefit.

RAMASWAMI: When you control a part of the body while you practice asana or pranayama, you may say that prana flows to that place. So when you say that prana flows to the naval when you do uddiyana bandha, it means that you are controlling that area by controlling the muscles in that area. Since accessibility of different internal organs, such as the uterus or stomach, is possible only by the ability to deftly control different groups of muscles, the capacity to direct prana to those areas is acquired by yogic practice.

DAVID: What is the relationship between the breath and the prana?

RAMASWAMI: Prana, according to my guru, remains in the heart region and removes the dross in the body by expiration. It draws pure air from outside to facilitate the proper functioning of the gastric fire (jatharagni) and thus extends the span of life. According to *datu pata* (the study of roots or stems of Sanskrit words), *prana* and *svasa*, which is normally translated as "breath," are synonymous. So, *prana* can mean breath force or life force. In usage, *prana* is the life force and *svasa* is the actual breathing function. *Prana vayu* is the air that is inhaled; in Tamil books, the term *prana vayu* is used to denote oxygen.

DAVID: It sounds like the prana directs the breath, causes inhalation and exhalation. Then again, calming the breath, with *dirga* (long) and *suksma* (subtle) breathing, seems to gather and center the dispersed prana. So, the breath and the life force are in some kind of symbiotic relationship, each affecting the other. Is it true?

RAMASWAMI: Yes.

DAVID: Krishnamacharya says that prana resides in the heart region. But sometimes we say that prana travels out to the senses and returns. Then again, when the obstacle called kundalini has been removed, we say the prana enters the *sushumna nadi* (spinal pathway) and rises. Would you clarify this a bit? Does it mean that at times the prana travels from the heart region through the nadis?

Also, would we say that prana is not part of prakriti (nature)? If so, then is not prana indentical with purusha (self/soul)? For what else is there? And prana cannot be a part of purusha because, as I understand it, purusha has no parts.

RAMASWAMI: Prana's position is the heart region but it extends through the nadis (pathways). Without the prana's movement, the sensations are not experienced. In fact, paralysis is said to be a malfunction or blockage of the prana and other *vayus* (vital energy).

One way of withdrawing from the external world is to draw the *prana sakthi* (power) inward rather than moving it outward as we do in our normal day-to-day life. As the yamas and niyamas tend to help to limit the person's contact with the external world to a minimum, Kundalini yogis also try drawing the prana inward. Thus, after the kundalini block has been removed, the prana is drawn into the sushumna nadi and made to merge in the sahasrara in the head. In such case the yogi is in a samadhi. It is also common for Hatha yogis to be able to draw the prana in this manner. In such a case of "trance," it is very difficult to wake the yogi from the trance while in the yogic-seated position. Even when you shake the yogi, he/she will not feel any sensation, as the prana has been drawn inward and secured in sahasrara. To a lesser degree, we may say that in deep sleep we do not hear sounds that we normally will hear, as the prana is residing in the heart and not extending outward through the nadis.

Life force is part of prakriti. Though this is not explicitly stated in the *Yoga Sutras*, it is taken for granted. As a rule, anything that is experienced is not purusha. Since the life force is experienced within us, it is part of prakriti. *Samkhya Karika*, a text on the twin philosophy of yoga, refers to the five forces (vayus) as general activity (vritti) of the chitta. Sloka (verse) 29 of *Samkhya Karika* clearly indicates that prana and other vayus are the general activities of antah karana, which is a derivative of prakriti.

In yoga, the second sutra of *Patanjala Yoga*, in which chitta vritti is mentioned, refers to the five kinds of special vrittis pertaining to each mind or person. They include direct perception, and wrong knowledge. They take place in our chitta—which I may translate here as "brain." These are special and we are normally aware of them. The chitta also has generalized functions (*samanya karana vrittis*) of maintaining life, which we may call "involuntary life functions." According to yogis/Samkhyas these are maintained by the five pranas.

DAVID: What is prana sanchara?

RAMASWAMI: *Sanchara* means "flow" or "movement." *San + chara* = "complete movement." Prana sanchara is the proper flow of prana force. According to Hatha yoga, if the nadis, which are the conduits of prana force, are filled with impurities, the prana sanchara is affected. Several cleaning methods, such as the nadi sodhana pranayama, facilitate the proper sanchara of prana.

DAVID: The breath is said to be a manifestation of the ultimate reality. If this is so, then, when the mind is with the breath, the mind is with ultimate reality. So, when we bring the mind to the breath in asana or pranayama, is it the same as bringing the mind to God?

RAMASWAMI: Some of the Upanishads mention that the breath is a manifestation of the ultimate reality, Brahman. The objective of this approach is to understand that everything that exists emanates from the ultimate reality and is not different from it. This view is different from that of yogis and Samkhyas, who say that breath is from prakriti but the self (purusha) is different from it. This view is against the nondualistic view of Advaita Vedantins.

DAVID: In HYP II, 15 we have another death threat (although my other translation uses the word "harm" in place of "kill"): the prana should be brought under control gradually, or else it will kill the practitioner. Is the prana so dangerous if we proceed with haste?

In the *sloka* (verse), it says it is so because the power of prana is compared to that of the lion, elephant, or tiger. Is it really so powerful? When I do my pranayama practice, I often feel the calming and quieting of the mind, but not this kind of power.

RAMASWAMI: Yes, when you do pranayama correctly (*vidhivat*), as Svatmarama says, all the positive results accrue. If you know how to swim, you can swim in water, but one who does not know how to swim drowns. Fire is helpful: it keeps us warm, cooks our food; but, out of control, it can destroy everything. A gentle breeze is pleasant, brings joy. But when the breeze becomes a tornado, it could be a big killer. If I say that one should take all safety measures when dealing with electricity, fire, or a tiger, am I scaring away people? So it is with correct pranayama practice. What Svatmarama says may be an exaggeration, but just as we warn a child to be careful with fire, a novice should be cautioned about improper practice, especially improper breath-holding.

✣ PREPARATION FOR PRANAYAMA ✣
INCLUDING KAPALABHATI

DAVID: A friend asks: "If I want to just do a pranayama practice, what is the minimal asana practice before pranayama? I ask this question because (a) sometimes I walk or bike in the morning instead of doing asanas; and (b) sometimes I have done an asana and pranayama practice in the morning, but in addition I would like to practice some pranayama in the afternoon."

RAMASWAMI: It again depends on individual needs and feeling. A good stretch routine of about fifteen minutes should be sufficient.

DAVID: Another friend writes: "I notice that if I do my kapalabhati too rapidly, I go into *bhastrika* (bellowslike) pranayama. Is this natural? Is bhastrika done at a more rapid rate?"

RAMASWAMI: Kapalabhati should be done at a pace that suits the individual, neither slow nor too rapid. Between 80 to 120 per minute is the pace that will be comfortable. While kapalabhati is a kriya, a cleansing process, bhastrika is a pranayama in which the breathing is regulated. Maybe you should practice Kapalabhati for short a duration several times. Lapsing into bhastrika-type breathing happens to many, but it is not natural.

DAVID: What are the parameters of kapalabhati? Once we are comfortable doing kapalabhati 108 times (with three different hasta vinyasas) should we be content with that? Or, are there times when we might do more?

RAMASWAMI: Doing kapalabhati 108 times is a good number to practice. Some days you may wish to do two rounds of 108 each. That should be sufficient. Doing too much kapalabhati could result in upsetting the chemical balance and, in some, produce giddiness. There are cases where excess kapalabhati has resulted in the weakening of the abdominal walls, resulting in herniation, whereas it is supposed to strengthen the abdominal walls. There is a staying in Tamil: "Even nectar in excess is poison."

DAVID: Another question: "I have been practicing kapalabhati and I find it very helpful. After two rounds of kapalabhati (54 times) followed by twelve pranayamas (5:5:10:5), I find I am calm, light, and peaceful. Should I repeat the exercise a second time?"

RAMASWAMI: In almost all my practice sessions with my teacher, he invariably used to ask me to end the session with a good round of kapalabhati followed by pranayama and finally a few minutes of shanmukhi mudra. I am glad you like the kapalabhati exercise. You may perhaps slowly increase it to 108 times. One round is sufficient. You may use different arms or hand positions for kapalabhati, for better and more varied effect.

DAVID: A follow-up question: "In building up to 108 kapalabhatis in one round (without a break), should I just keep adding 10 or 20 more kapalabhatis to my first round. For example, should I do 64 kapalabhatis the first round, rest, and then do 44 on the second round to equal a total of 108? Or, should I just do one round and keep adding to it?"

RAMASWAMI: You may start with 36. Then add another 36 and finally 36 more to reach the magical figure of 108. I would even suggest that you change the position of the arms/hands for the three 36s. While teaching, one may start around 24 and keep increasing at increments of 12.

DAVID: What is a good age to begin teaching kapalabhati to children, and what should follow this kriya?

RAMASWAMI: Kapalabhati is a very good preliminary kriya to practicing pranayama. As, in the olden days, children were initiated into Vedic studies at the age of five, and pranayama was a part of the daily ritual, age five or seven should be okay for children. But children tend to hold the breath playfully or do more than the recommended times of kapalabhati because of curiosity, so instead I would suggest that kapalabhati be started at the age of about twelve or thirteen, when they can be expected to be more careful. Just as asanas exercise the body, kapalabhati and pranayama help to exercise the respiratory system, the internal muscles, and the internal organs. These respiratory exercises are very useful. But considerable caution should be exercised because children are children.

132

✵ FOCUS OF MIND ✵

DAVID: If I suggest that the mind follow the breath in pranayama, where is the mind focused when holding or suspending the breath (kumbhaka)?

If I have the student count the breath, then the mind can also count during the kumbhaka and stay that way. Similarly, if we do pranayama with mantra, then the mantra is repeated during hold and the mind stays with that.

RAMASWAMI: What you say is correct. Actually, the pranayama mantra is recited during hold in the classical "with-mantra pranayama." Since there are a definite number of syllables, and a definite time duration of each syllable, it is sufficient to just chant the mantra during hold, whereas the inhalation and exhalation may have to be timed by rhythmic counting. The necessity to count during hold comes when you do pranayama without a definite mantra.

Many people do not care to use the mantra; still, you can hold the breath without the mantra or counting. Over a period of time, the practitioner is able to hold the breath for a predefined time. During that time, he/she may watch the pranasthana (the place where breathing appears to be centered in the chest), or sometimes the middle of the eyebrows (or different chakras in the body). Of course, when first starting out these practices are best learned from a teacher.

DAVID: The pranasthana moves up and down (also left and right?) from day to day and even during the course of one day. What is the significance of this? Is it saying something about the location of prana? Something about the quality of prana? Something about the flow of prana?

RAMASWAMI: In chapter 2, I explained the pranasthana in an empirical manner. Prana is said to move downward in internal holding of breath, and apana is said to move up in mula and uddiyana bandhas. When a yogi is able to achieve the union of these two, then it is yoga. One definition of yoga is the union of prana and apana.

DAVID: If we say prana resides in the heart, then is the pranasthana the same as the heart? And, does "heart" mean the place the emotions appear to emanate from, and not the physical heart?

RAMASWAMI: Pranasthana is the spot or center, inside the chest, from where breathing appears to start and into which exhalation appears to converge. The practitioner can find this empirical spot by close observation.

DAVID: I still have trouble holding the mind on the breath and the pranasthana. My mind keeps jumping around, to the events of the day, to what I'm going to eat, or other distractions.

RAMASWAMI: If the mind likes the practice, it will settle down. If there is effort and struggle, it will not.

DAVID: I have a question on *dristi*, where to fix the attention during asana and pranyama. Sometimes we watch the pranasthana, sometimes the place between the eyebrows, sometimes one of the other chakras. Does each have a different effect? How do we choose? Or, should this be learned from a teacher?

RAMASWAMI: Usually, during pranayama, it will be useful to focus attention in the pranasthana, so that the expansion of chest is uniform and also to obviate the tendency, normally experienced by untrained people, to tighten the chest muscles. While practicing dharana (concentration), however, Patnjali suggests focusing at one place (YS III, 1). Vyasa, in his commentary, gives a number of spots, inside the body, to focus one's attention on, such as: *nabhichakra* (navel or manipuraka chakra), *hrudayapundarika* (heart lotus/anahata chakra), *murdhni jyotoshi* (light in the head, Agna chakra), *nasikagra* (beginning of the nose), or *jihvagra* (beginning/tip of the tongue). Also suggested are places outside the body or outside objects (such as the icon of the favorite deity, or others). Later on in the third chapter of YS, several sidhhis are said to be achieved when the yoga practitioner is able to convert the dharana into a samyama (complete concentration).

So, the object of focus should be determined by what one is easily able to focus on. This can be decided by the student with the help of the teacher. In the initial stages, it will be appropriate to choose a sthana, a place to start dharana. Once you are able to do samyama on one place or object, such as a chakra, then the yogi will be able to focus on other objects or places. Thereby, he/she will be able to do samyama on subtler and different objects and, by applying the same procedure, will be able to attain different siddhis (see YS III, 6).

DAVID: In YY V, 17–20 (I'm following Mohan's translation), Yajnavalkya gives his instructions on the technique of Nadishodana to his wife, Gargi. Here, he recommends meditating on the fire in the belly during the practice. Does it make a great difference in the results if we are meditating on a different object?

RAMASWAMI: According to Patanjali, one of the parameters to be considered in the practice of pranayama is *desa*, a place where you want to focus your attention. In this case, Yagnyavalkya recommends that attention be directed to the belly. This place is the position of jatharagni (gastric fire). At the end of inhalation the chest is full and the diaphragm is pushed down and it is easy to focus on the mid-part of the body, the belly. The ideation is that the jatharagni traverses upward, and the prana vayu drawn in during inhalation and held in kumbhaka increases the intensity of gastric fire. And, the *agni bijakshara* mantra is used.

135

Pranayama done with mantra is called *samantraka pranayama*. Sometimes it is also called *sagarbha pranayama*, especially when some bhavana or meditation, such as the gastric fire as in this case, is used.

Thus we see that, depending on the stage of the pranayama, different desa come into play. If you do mula bandha, after exhalation, the attention will be directed to the rectal region (muladhara). The type of pranayama and the stage of the pranayama will determine where you will direct your attention.

DAVID: In commenting on YS I, 34, *pracchardana vidharanabhyam* (complete expulsion of breath and holding the breath out), Hariharananda Aranya (a modern commentator on YS) makes the point that, for it to become calm, the mind needs to hold on to something. In fact, he goes on, if we practice pranayama without dhyana (meditation), the mind will become more disturbed instead of calm. Do you agree with this? That letting the mind wander during pranayama will not only be ineffective, but will cause more harm than good?

RAMASWAMI: Yes, it is absolutely right. There is a saying, "The mind is unstable and fickle." In fact, all the methods suggested in this section, starting from YS I, 34, urge the practitioner to use one practice that basically is one-pointedness.

Pranayama without dhyana or any bhavana is called *agarbha pranayama*, and several yoga texts say that this kind of practice is inferior. Therefore in the scheme of vinyasa krama, as taught by my guru, the use of breath even during asana practice helps to bring the mind under considerable control. Unfortunately, many schools teach yoga without the use of breath, saying that breath control will be done in pranayama. But then they seldom teach pranayama. In the Vinyasa krama, some breathing control is introduced in asana practice. And, in pranayama practice some dhyana is introduced.

Samantraka pranayama (pranayama with mantra), helps to focus the mind. I do not think it is possible to do pranayama without attending to the breath. Of course, there are some people who do a few long inhalations and exhalations and call it pranayama, without adhering to the various parameters such as the place, time, duration, and others mentioned in the *Yoga Sutras*. But once one scrupulously follows all the parameters in pranayama, it is difficult to do it without attention.

❦ ALIGNMENT ❧

DAVID: How much can we rely on proper breathing to automatically bring about correct alignment?

RAMASWAMI: First the alignment and then proper breathing. If the pranayama breathing is not free or is impaired you may, to some extent, correct it by proper alignment, facilitated by proper yogic posture such as the lotus and vajrasana. The hip and shoulder joints are important and should be sufficiently flexible so that the spine can be pulled up. Jalandhara bandha also stretches the spine, especially the thoracic spine. With these, postural impediments to breathing can be overcome. Then of course the nadis that conduct the prana also should be cleaned. This can be achieved by such kriyas as kapalbhati, and pranayama as nadi sodhana.

✿ STOPPING THE BREATH ✿

DAVID: In HYP II, 9, it is suggested that we hold after inhale, as long as possible, until we are covered with perspiration or the body shakes. Isn't this extreme? I thought the most important thing was to be comfortable in pranayama. Of course, the sloka (verse) does go on to say the exhale needs to be slow. Perhaps this requirement serves to moderate the hold after inhale. Or, could this sloka be about a kriya for cleansing the nadis and not technically pranayama?

RAMASWAMI: This sloka should be read with the previous two verses. The yoga practitioner, after mastering a yogic posture, say, the lotus, should do pranayama as the author suggests. Here he suggests, to start with, holding the breath to the extent that one can. It may be a couple of seconds or even more. Then, in the sloka under reference, he says that one should hold the breath more, or longer, to one's capacity, but should be able to exhale smoothly and continue further with pranayama. Brahmananda, taking a cue from subsequent slokas, suggests that one should hold until one starts sweating.

We can see that this is a gradual process. First, practice kumbhaka consistently per your capacity and then extend the hold, thereby improving the vital holding capacity. In the initial stages, when you try to hold the breath for a longer period of time, there could be some discomfort, and you may start sweating. At that point, stop the hold and exhale slowly. For many people, breathholding is uncomfortable. Some even panic. Many people do not take to swimming for fear of inhaling while in water, fear of uncoordinated breathing. In my classes, when I teach pranayama, more than half do not do the breathing as prescribed. I have had students come up at the end of a pranayama session and say that holding the breath, especially after exhalation, creates panic in them. They are afraid that even a moment more of holding the breath will result in dizziness. Many yoga teachers are, themselves, not comfortable with pranayama, and they conveniently skip the seemingly innocuous pranayama practice.

138   The yogi should be able to do pranayama following definite parameters, such as the 1:4:2 ratio. In samantra pranayama, it is found that you need to hold the breath for at least 20 seconds during every one of a number of successive pranayamas. How can one get the capacity of complete control over all the aspects of breathing without correct practice? We should understand that even as pranayama is within the capacity of everyone to do, and it has immense benefits, it should be learned and practiced slowly and deliberately. Everyone knows that a tiger or an elephant or a lion can be tamed, but one has to have the training and also follow correct procedures. Just as a novice cannot tame a tiger, a novice cannot do pranayama properly.

DAVID: HYP II, 13 suggests rubbing the perspiration (arising from pranayama) into the body, saying this brings strength and lightness. But surely it is the pranayama that gives these qualities, not our sweat.

RAMASWAMI: Again, here we have to see the context. Perspiration is common in the early stages of pranayama practice, as Svatmarama says. Normally, to keep the body hot, we wipe the perspiration away with a towel because the perspiration produced by the anxious pranayama practitioner is to reduce the heat. So what Svatmarama suggests is to make use of the sweatiness of the skin to massage one's own body with the moisture. The massage will be easier to do with a wet skin than a dry skin. It will help to relax the tense muscles.

My guru used to ask us to have regular oil baths. One should massage by oneself. He would say, "Don't allow someone else to touch and massage your body." I, as a yogi, know my body better and I should be the one to do it. Such massaging helps to relax the muscles, improves blood circulation (*ratka sanchara*). So, for the yogi who has just started on pranayama, the massage could be very helpful. Later on, when he/she has mastered the practice of pranayama, going beyond the stages of perspiring and trembling, he/she gets all the qualities you have said.

139

DAVID: "*Cale vate calam cittam*" (HYP II, 2)—When the breath stops so does the mind. Is the meaning that we literally stop the breath? Or, is it that we make the flow very smooth and evenly, dirga and sukshma? Is this similar to YS II, 51, where some say "stopping the breath," and others interpret it differently?

RAMASWAMI: The word *cala*, even as it means "to move," has, generally, a negative connotation. It is used to indicate trembling, shaking, agitation, unfixedness, wavy movement. So when the author says *cale*—that is, when the movement of *vate* (breath), is unsteady—then the mind also is fickle and unsteady. It merely indicates a correlation. The word *nischala* is more an evenness of the breath, than the cessation of movement of breath. But, YS II, 51 indicates stoppage of breath, or kumbhaka. Some interpret the stoppage as occurring at random, and some say it indicates stoppage after exhalation (bahya kumbhaka)

DAVID: In HYP II, 71 and 72, the *sahita* (with breathing) and *kevala* (breath-holding only) kumbhaka are described. What is the difference between these two? The text talks as though there were no inhale or exhale involved in kevala kumbhanka. Is this then the same as when some speak of stopping the breath in YS II, 51?

RAMASWAMI: When you do kumbhaka preceded by deliberate inhalation (puraka) and followed by exhalation, it is sahita breath-holding (sahita kumbhaka). If you suddenly hold the breath at any moment, without deep inhalation and exhalation to follow as in classical pranayama, it is called kevala kumbhaka. The capacity to hold breath without the help of inhalation and exhalation indicates a high degree of proficiency in pranayama (pranayama or kumbhaka siddhi).

140

DAVID: We say that long inhale and exhale in asana prepare for pranayama. But, Patanjali defines pranayama as kumbhaka. So, how does this help?

RAMASWAMI: According to Hatha yogis, breath-holding is the important aspect when the prana-apana merger takes place. But we have to do the sahita kumbhaka to be able to do kevala kumbhaka. Since the goal is kumbhaka, pranayama is also called kumbhaka. Actually, one meaning of the term *pranayama* is to hold the breath. *Pranasya aayamah*, or holding of the breath is pranayama. One of the meanings of the word *aayaama* is "to restrain, to stop."

DANGERS

DAVID: In the commentary to HYP I, 16, we are warned that we may finish our lives as maniacs or suicides if we practice pranayama without first establishing yama niyama. Is the purpose here to scare me into following the proper practice? If so, he has succeeded.

RAMASWAMI: One of the important lessons of pranayama is that the breath, and hence the mind, can be brought under voluntary control. But we also know that improper breath-holding efforts by ordinary people could lead to problems. Children sometimes compete among themselves trying to find out who can hold the breath longest, and sometimes end up becoming dizzy or even unconscious. Since breathing is a very important physiological function, which could affect the supply of oxygen to the brain, one has to be quite cautious while practicing breathing exercises. Pranayama is more delicate than the practice of asanas. Mistakes in practice of asanas are generally not as calamitous as mistakes in pranayama.

Yogis found the correct method to use the breath to control the mind and improve health; whereas improper interference with breathing, including long breath-holding without preparatory aspects, such as diaphragmatic exercises, proper inhalations and exhalations, and conditioning of the thoracic muscles and the intercostal muscles, could be harmful. That improper interference with the breath can affect the mind is the view of yogis and even modern medicine. Yes, it is not merely to scare one to follow the correct procedure, but also to indicate the real danger of improper practice.

141

❦ MODULATED BREATH ❧

DAVID: What is meant by modulated breath?

RAMASWAMI: Just as a singer modulates the voice, the yogic breathing also will require very good control and variation. In vinyasa krama yoga practice and in pranayama, we are required to synchronize the breathing with the movements and do controlled breathing for different durations of time. The yogi should have total control over breathing while practicing vinyasa krama yoga and also while doing the different varieties of pranayama. In all these, the breathing should be smooth and, equally important, uniform. That is, the flow of air should be uniform. Many people, while doing yogic breathing exercises, will inhale with a start, sometimes as if gasping. We should be able to vary the rate of flow of air, depending upon the length of the breath, but still the flow of air should be smooth and uniform. What I mean by modulating the breath are these factors: Yoga texts give examples of how the inhalations and exhalations should be. While inhaling, it should be *nilothphala nalavath*, as smooth as drinking water through the stem of a blue water lily. Just as when you drink water through a straw, it has uniform flow, so should be the flow of air. The exhalation should be like *taila dharavath*, or the flow of poured oil. When oil is poured from a ladle, it has a uniform flow, unlike water, which is not viscous.

❧ ANULOMA AND VILOMA ❧

DAVID: In YR II, 49 the practices of *anuloma* and *viloma* (with and against the grain) krama are mentioned. What are the uses of these?

RAMASWAMI: Let me first explain what these different pranayamas are. Normally, ujjayi breathing is throat breathing, in and out. The three kramas usually associated with ujjayi pranayama are its variants. For these, three prefixes are added to the word *loma*. *Anu* means "to follow" or "in line with," as in *anusasana* in the *Yoga Sutras*. The prefix *prati* implies "opposing, counter to," as in *pratipaksha* or *pratikriya*. The prefix *vi* would indicate "variety," as in *vinyasa*. The word *loma* means "hair." In a lighter vein, I may say that if one shaves with a downward stroke, it is *anuloma* because the movement is in the direction of the hair growth. If one shaves with upward strokes, against the grain as it were, it will be *pratiloma*, and if one uses both the strokes, say, downward over the cheeks and upward over the chin, that is variety, *viloma*.

So in ujjayi pranayama, when one inhales through the throat and exhales through one nostril, then it is anuloma. It is so because the flow of air is in the direction of the bristles in the nostril (assuming the hair grows downward). If the individual inhales through right nostril, exhales through the throat, and repeats it with the left nostril as well, it will be pratiloma ujjayi, because the flow of air in the nostril is against the direction of the hair. Now, if one would inhale through the right nostril and exhale through throat, then inhale through throat and exhale through left, then inhale through left to exhale through throat, followed by a throat inhalation with exhalation through the right nostril, then one would complete one cycle of viloma ujjayi, because the airflow in the nostrils is both in the direction of the hair and also against the grain. There are a few more variations, such as interrupted inhalations, but suffice it to say that there are many different varieties of pranayama. The parameters of pranayama include the place of control, the time duration of each phase of pranayamic breathing, the number of times the pranayama is done, which mantra is used, when the mantra is used, and whether pranayama is done with the bandhas or without them. These are the important ones.

143

What are the benefits of this variety of pranayamas? Just as the vinyasa krama helps to create a comprehensive workout for the whole system, the variety of pranayamas help to bring better control over the entire breathing apparatus. For instance, in the case of the loma group of pranayama vinyasas, we have a hybrid kind of pranayama, combining the ujjayi and nadisodhana, thereby reaping the benefits of both pranayamas.

1:4:2

DAVID: In YR II, 59, the pranayama ratio of 1:4:2 is spoken of as special. Is this ratio risky? Who can do it?

RAMASWAMI: In fact, almost all yoga texts mention or detail this particular pranayama. Because of the preponderance of antah kumbhak for a disproportionately long period, many people shy away from this pranayama. The ratio you refer to is one time unit of inhalation, four time units of holding the breath, and two time units of exhalation.

Normally, we breathe at the rate of about fifteen times per minute. Our inhalation and exhalations are usually for about 2 seconds each. So if you introduce this ratio, keeping the inhalation at about 2 seconds, you will have to hold the breath for about 8 seconds, and take 4 seconds for exhalation. In this manner, you will do just about four breaths per minute as opposed to fifteen breaths per minute. Of course, one who is uninitiated can do it once or twice, but if required to do it for a number times in succession, he/she may find it difficult to maintain the ratio. Many people find the exhalation swift and uncontrollable after the long breath-holding.

This ratio is used in mantra pranayama. There are a few well-known mantras, such as the Vedic pranayama mantra and the "siva-siva" mantra. The Vedic pranayama mantra, consisting of sixty-four syllables (matras), takes about 20 seconds to chant mentally. According to several texts, including *Manu Smriti* (classic on Hindu way of life), the mantra is to be chanted while holding in the breath. So one should be able to hold the breath for 20 seconds, during which time the mantra is chanted. If so, with the 1:4:2 ratio, the inhalation has to be 5 seconds and the exhalation 10 seconds. It will thus take about 35 seconds, and if you take a 5-second bahya kumbhaka, then it could be about 40 to 45 seconds. It is the normal practice in Vedic pranayama to do at least ten rounds in one sitting, which would mean that the practitioner should be able to sit in a yogic posture steadily for this duration and do the pranayamas without losing control. If you go by the *Hatha Yoga Pradipika*, one can go up to eighty pranayamas at a stretch. This would mean that one has to sit in a posture for about an hour and do pranayama and follow the ratios correctly, without panicking or without discomfort. Some texts suggest holding out the breath for 20 seconds, especially texts of Hatha yogis and Kundalini yogis.

My one-to-one studies with my guru usually lasted one hour. One day, at the beginning of the class, he asked me to do this pranayama for the entire duration of the session and left the room. At the end of one hour he walked in to the room, asked me to join the end-of-the-session peace invocation, and left the room. He did not say anything, but looked pleased. There were many other occasions when he asked me to devote the entire session to pranayama.

It is sad that yoga students seldom practice pranayama and that contemporary teachers appear to have disdain for pranayama. It is a very important and a very useful aspect of yoga. Pranayama reduces tamas or darkness and increases satwa or clarity.

145

SITALI

DAVID: If I am a *vata* type, often cold and nervous, does that mean it would be incorrect for me to practice sitali pranayama (a breathing exercise), often regarded as a cooling pranayama? (Of course, I could make sitali more brmhana [brahmana] by holding after inhale or visualizing the sun, but the basic pranayama is, I think, supposed to be cooling.) And, is it the same for chandra bhedana?

RAMASWAMI: I am not an expert on Ayurveda. I think a *kapha* (phlegm) person should not take cold things. Anyway, if something is contraindicated, as a general principle, for a person, it does not mean that it applies to him/her at all times. So a kapha person may find sitali pranayama very useful when the weather is very warm, or when some cooling to the system will be needed.

NADI SHODANA

DAVID: A friend writes, "I do my yoga practice in the morning, usually around 8:00 AM. The end of my asana practice is followed by kapalabhati (108 times). I have tried to do nadi shodhana following kapalabhati, but no matter what variations I use with my kapalabhati (arm positions or using one nasal passage and then the other) I cannot achieve a pleasant-feeling nadi shodhana (especially with kumbhaka) due to nasal blockage. (My ujjayi pranayamas are performed with ease at 5:5:10:5.) However, if I try nadi shodhana at noon, it is okay—my nadis are open at that time of day. Since my practice is in the morning, I have eliminated nadi sodhana from my practice. Is that okay? And, what should be the next step in my pranayama practice?

RAMASWAMI: If you are not comfortable with nadi sodhana in the morning but can do ujjayi, you may practice ujjayi in the morning and later on, if you find time, can do nadi shodhana. The nasal congestion in the mornings can be due to some minor allergic reaction resulting in secretions which tend to swell the nostrils. Perhaps you may try staying for a longer period of time in sarvangasana (or viparita karani), in your asana practice. Sarvangasana helps retain blood circulation to the head and face and may help relieve congestion. If you have some deviation of septum, then also minor congestion of the nostrils could create some problem. The next step will be to stay in shanmukhi mudra for a longer time and see if you are able to remain with the breath during this period.

☙ BHASTRIKA KUMBHAKA ☙

DAVID: In HYP III, 115, bhastrika kumbhaka is talked about for rousing the kundalini. Is the idea here to take a certain number of rapid exhalations and then follow this with an inhalation and a hold after inhale? Is this bhastrika kumbhaka ever used in vinyasa krama?

RAMASWAMI: This sloka should be read with the previous few slokas in which the preparations for moving the kundalini and the nature of kandasthana are explained. Bhastrika, with its bellows-like movement, helps to move the kundalini; kapalabhati could be equally effective.

My teacher had explained bhastrika, but kapalabhati used to be the exercise of choice for him. That was what he used to ask me to do.

147

✸ PLAVINI ✸

DAVID: In HYP II, 70, the pranayama called plavini (a type of pranayama emphasizing inhale) is mentioned. Does this involve a long hold after inhale? Is this the pranayama that was thought to lead to levitation? In the text, it states that the yogin floats over deep water like a lotus leaf.

RAMASWAMI: The word *plavana* means "to float, sail over" or "leap." So as the name of the pranayama indicates, this particular procedure helps one to "float."

I was never interested in the siddhis, nor did my teacher show any inclination to teach me any of the siddhis. However, I would like to mention that to watch the way my teacher used to do pranayama was, in itself, a great experience. He would do nadi shodhana smoothly for a long time. The chest would expand like a balloon, like a rubber balloon. The expansion of his chest would be phenomenal. I once had to resist the temptation of asking him if I could use a measuring tape to meter his chest expansion. And after nadi shodhana, he would do kumbhaka without any discomfort whatsoever.

So plavini is a special kind of pranayama in which puraka (inhalation) plays an important role. There is also an interesting story about Hanuman, or Anjaneya, leaping over the Indian Ocean to reach Lanka. *Ramayana* narrates vividly the procedure adapted by Anjaneya to leap over the ocean. He went up a hill, did deep pranayama, and, holding his breath, leapt over the ocean like a glider or hovercraft.

❧ PRANAYAMA AND THE BANDHAS ❧

DAVID: In YR I, 67 it says the uddiyana bandha (abdominal lock) is the basis for jalandhara bandha (chin lock) (figure 3-1). What is meant by this? Are they related to each other through the spine?

RAMASWAMI: Rigidity of the hip joints is one of the main causes of problems with the spine. Classic yoga postures such as padmasana and vajrasana help to relieve the tightness in the hip joint. Vajrasana especially, by supporting the buttocks bones with the heels and the arch formed by the ankle and the dorsum, is a very spine-friendly asana. So, the first step will be to choose a correct posture. In pasmasana, raising the arms slowly and stretching the sides is *parvatasana* (hill pose). In this, the spine is stretched and, to some extent, the hip joint loosens so that you can stretch the spine and also pull up the pelvis by stretching the hip joints as well. Now, in the same pose, after a complete exhalation, if you contract the glutei (rectum), and pull up the pelvic floor, you will be doing mula bandha. Then, if, in a continuous motion, you draw the abdomen inward and backward, you have the two bandhas, mula and uddiyana. By raising the pelvic floor in mula bandha, you are able to pull up the hip joint from inside. With the hip joint freed, it becomes easier to keep the back erect and do the jalandhara bandha by stretching the cervical spine. Here, the capacity to do a very powerful mula bandha is facilitated by a correct pose, as is the capacity to empty the lungs as completely as possible. Please see the picture of my guru doing the three bandhas in a posture on page 80 of *Yoga Rahasya*, July 1998 edition. My teacher used to say that most of the benefits of yoga can be achieved by the capacity for strength of exhalation (*recaka bala*). Good recaka is a prerquisite of powerful mula and uddiyana bandhas.

So, to answer the question, yes.

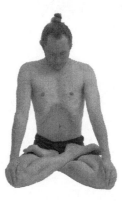

149

Figure 3-1

DAVID: YR I, 95 states that pranayama done without the bandhas is useless. Not only that, but it may allow all types of diseases. Is this possible? If I give some simple breathing (without bandhas) to a class, is there really some danger to this?

RAMASWAMI: I think there is a slight variation that has crept into the printed text. The last but one word in the sloka should be *aaspada* and not *aspada*, as seen in the printed version. I checked my handwritten notes. In that case, the sloka may be translated as follows: "That pranayama which is done without the three bandhas will be without the (intended) benefits. So no independent (without bandha) practice of pranayama is recommended. The body will be an abode of all diseases."

I think the translation that the practice of pranayama without bandhas may produce diseases is far-fetched. I think the import of the sloka is to encourage the practice of pranayama with the bandhas. It implies that practice of pranayama alone, without the bandhas, may not produce the desired results; it will not be helpful in the prevention and eradication of the diseases.

As the footnote suggests, the teacher and the practitioner should slowly introduce the practice of bandhas, after successfully mastering any pranayama. I feel that the sloka mainly emphasizes the importance of the bandha practice. As I have mentioned elsewhere, yoga is a *sarvanga sadhana*, a practice for all parts of the body, including or especially the internal organs, the main kosas—the heart, lungs, stomach, large intestines, bladder, and uterus/prostate. These internal organs can be accessed only by the three bandhas. And the three bandhas can be effectively practiced only by complete exhalation (rechaka), which requires that all the parameters of pranayama, inhalation, exhalation, and breath-holding in and out, should be very good. Since all of them are interrelated, for the complete benefit of yoga is to be obtained, both pranayama and bandhas should be mastered. Simple yogic breathing exercises are quite useful for the beginning yoga practitioner.

DAVID: Is the practice of bandhas going to disturb my sleep? Will it disturb my bowel and urinary functions? (YR III, 14).

RAMASWAMI: This particular sloka should be read with reference to the context. It refers to yoga during pregnancy. Kapalabhati and bhastrika, being powerful lower abdominal movements, are contraindicated during pregnancy. These are active and energizing functions, and could disturb the sleep of the rather taut pregnant woman. Because of the pelvic pressure already existing in this condition, additional pressures induced by the powerful pelvic floor movements of kapalabhati/bhastrika could affect the pelvic organs such as the bladder, and also the large intestine. This sloka is not meant for the general yoga practitioner who could derive considerable benefits by the practice of kapalabhati. I have also explained the technique and the benefits of kapalabhati in my book, *Yoga for the Three Stages of Life*, pages 190–94.

DAVID: In the practice of mula and uddiyana bandhas after exhale, does it matter in which order they are done? That is, can we draw in and lift the navel followed by lifting the rectum just as well as lifting the rectum first, and then drawing the navel in and up? Also, following hold after exhale, should one release uddiyana and sustain mula through the next inhale, or release both?

RAMASWAMI: I have found that doing the mula bandha first, and then uddiyana bandha, is easier and natural. Mula bandha also helps to loosen the hip and the pelvic floor, so that later it can be lifted up in uddiyana bandha. Some schools suggest keeping the mula bandha continually, but in vinyasa krama practice, treating both the bandhas together is easier. It also helps to work on the rectal muscles repeatedly.

151

DAVID: In HYP III, 73, Svatmarama says that jalandhara bandha controls the sixteen *adharas* (vital centers). These range from the toes up to the skull. So, Jalandhara bandha is affecting the entire body. How does this happen? Is this because jalandhara bandha closes ida and pingala nadis and so controls the flow of prana throughout the whole body?

RAMASWAMI: The default position of the head in vinyasa krama is to be in jalandhara bandha, or at least a head-down position. One reason is that it facilitates slow, smooth, synchronized breathing with the movements in the vinyasa method of asana practice.

My teacher used to maintain chin lock during all the postures, except when there was a particular reason to change. You may check some of his old pictures to confirm this. In chaturanga-dandasana, and even in urdhva-mukha swanasana (upward-facing dog position), he would hold the head in jandhara bandha, if he were to stay in the pose for several breaths.

The author of *Nyaya Sutras* (the sutras of a Vedic philosophy), Gowtama, was also known as Akshipada, because he kept his head down and his gaze was at his feet (*Akshi* = eyes, *pada* = foot).

The chin-down position has the important effect of stretching the spine. The way to stretch your spine is to keep your head down, pull up the waist, and stretch the backbone. This is not possible if you keep the head straight, which will only hamper the upward movement of the spine.

When the spine is stretched and kept straight, it facilitates the movement of prana (and kundalini) along the sushumna. Since all the pranas are to be drawn from the peripheries of the body inward, jalandhara bandha has a definite place in yoga practice. While maha mudra, mula and uddiyana bandhas, such kriyas as kapalabhati, or bhastrika pranayama all work on the pelvic and abdominal areas, jalandhara bandha helps to keep the spine erect to facilitate the flow of kundalini/prana up and through the chakras easily.

152

❧ SIDDHASANA ❧

DAVID: HYP I, 42 states that when siddhasana is mastered, the three bandhas follow without effort and naturally. What is the meaning here? Surely we still have to apply some effort to master the bandhas.

RAMASWAMI: You can see that siddhasana (figure 3-2) helps to laterally stretch the pelvic muscles extensively. Furthermore, the posture opens the hip joints to almost ninety degrees. These two help to create sufficient space for the rectal muscles and the pelvic floor to move more easily. "Without effort" should be interpreted as "effortlessly" or "easily."

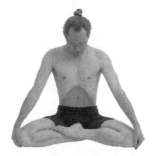

Figure 3-2

❧ NAULI ❧

DAVID: Was *nauli* (an abdominal cleansing practice) (figure 3-3) taught by Krishnamacharya? Or was this one of the kriyas he considered unnecessary? In HYP II, 34 it is referred to as the crown of Hatha yoga practice.

RAMASWAMI: My guru has written about nauli in his book *Yoga Makaranda.* He taught nauli, but did not emphasize it in the same way as he would the three bandhas. Among kriyas, his favorite was kapalabhati.

Nauli is a very powerful abdominal exercise indeed. He used a procedure very similar to nauli to relieve tightness of the stomach. He would isolate, then hold the rectus abdominus of the patient and gently pull it and release it. The tightness would vanish.

In relation to this, I have described an experience I had with my teacher in my book *Yoga for the Three Stages of Life* (page 7).

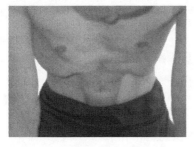

Figure 3-3

❧ UTGHATA ❧

DAVID: What is *utghata* (opening of the gate)? And, what is its role in pranayama?

RAMASWAMI: Brahmananda, while writing a commentary of the *Hatha Yoga Pradipika* of Svatmarama, interprets the word *Hatha* as being "pranayama." *Ha* is "prana" and *tha* is "apana," and the integration of these two is Hatha yoga. According to him, the principal means of achieving the goal of Hatha yoga is pranayama. What are the principal steps involved? First, the Hatha yogi will carefully isolate him/herself from the distractions and disturbances of the external word and also unhealthy personal habits by a conscious practice and observances of yama niyamas until they become habitual (samskara). One will also practice some of the kriyas to cleanse the nadis, mentioned in Hatha yoga texts. Then one will diligently practice the required asanas mentioned in the Hatha yoga texts and thereby prepare one's body to be fit to practice the higher Hatha yoga. One will practice pranayama, especially the kumbhakas. Even here, one will practice very long, complete, and smooth exhalation and be able to remain in external breath holding (bahya kumbhaka). Why does one want this? That is how one can do rectal and abdominal locks (mula bandha and uddiyana bandha) well and in a sustained manner. According to Hatha yogis, the mula bandha helps to push the apana up, and then it can unite with prana with the help of uddiyana bandha. My guru used to say that everything could be achieved by the efficacy of yogic exhalation. This united prana is close to the position of fire (jatharagni), which heats the prana. Once the prana is thus heated up, and pushed back by the Bandhas, it disturbs the dormant, coiled kundalini. Because of the sustained blockage of other nadis by mula and uddiyana bandhas, the awakened kundalini is forced to enter the spine (sushumna) and travel upward, cutting through the nerve hubs (chakras) and knots (*granthis*). It rushes up the spine and finally opens sahasrara, for ultimate merger with Siva and subsequent release (moksha). This opening of the gate, as it were, is called utghata, like flinging open the door after opening the door with the correct key. It is similar to a man coming out of a manhole, pushing up the manhole cover with effort. So pranayama becomes the key means of attaining the ultimate goal, which the Hatha yogis also call moksha. I remember my guru saying once, in connection with utghata, that sometimes one feels a substantial blow of the head from inside while practicing pranayama.

So after the yogi is able to achieve utghata, the whole yogic "heaven" is open to him/her. He/she lives the rest of his life in this great samadhi. Ultimately, when he/she passes away, the prana will go out through the Brahmarandhra (some yogis relate it to the area of anterior fontanelle, the soft area of the head seen in infants). In olden times, the belief was that, depending upon how the prana finally departs, one can know to which "world" the dead person would go. While the yogi gets the prana released as mentioned, lesser mortals would breathe out through the other nine orifices (nava dwara) of the body. The last breath could be through the mouth, the eyes, the nose, or even the anus. The gateway indicates the world one would go to! Sometimes this belief is taken to limits. When yogis or sanyasins die, they are kept in a yogic-seated posture and lowered into a pit. Then someone would smash a coconut on top of the head and make a crevice in the head indicating symbolically that the prana left the body by the "head" path.

But pranayama is not practiced merely for the kundalini arousal, as done by the Hatha yogis. Raja yogis use pranayama for the removal of tamas so that their citta can become fit for samyama, which is a process of the mind. Let me put it like this: The Hatha yogi's moksha is a physiological release, whereas the Raja yogis use pranayama so that the citta becomes very pure and able to realize the true nature of the self. For Raja yogis, moksha is the freedom of the mind.

Talking of *Hatha Yoga Pradipika*, my guru once said that there were no great *tatwas* (eternal principles) discussed in *Hatha Yoga*, implying that *Yoga Sutras* and other philosophical works will alone make us understand the eternal principles.

✺ SECRECY ✺

DAVID: In HYP I, 11 it is suggested that we keep the yoga secret, that it is ineffective when revealed. And, in Brahmananda's commentary, he states that everything is not revealed and the most important methods must be learned from a teacher. Without a teacher the student will come to harm. Did Krishnamacharya keep some knowledge secret? We have no way of knowing. Was pranayama once kept secret?

RAMASWAMI: Even now, it is well nigh impossible to practice pranayama correctly without proper initiation, proper instructions, and follow-up. It is very difficult to put into words several of the methods of yoga practice. Such exercises as sarvangasana and sirsasana were seldom explained in detail in the olden texts. Can a book explain all that is to be known about singing, painting, acting, or games?

I feel that my guru was willing to teach everything if he found or felt the student was willing and competent. If every guru keeps holding back something, the subject will die because every following generation will know less and less. And the lack of knowledge could be filled with innovations of novices, leading to corruption or the art itself dying. It is a matter of expediency that serious students should have a good teacher to guide them. Teachers of every generation should pass on the ancient knowledge to their students and not hold back from deserving students. Passing on the knowledge faithfully and diligently is the duty of every teacher of ancient sciences like yoga.

4

On Meditation

INTRODUCTION

WHY DO YOU want to meditate? It is a common buzzword. It relieves tension. It makes the mind relaxed and positive. My mind becomes clearer after some meditation. I sleep well. Yes, these are positive results that accrue to the practitioner, but they are not the only benefits. According to ancients, meditation is a process that transforms the mind for the better. A mind that is habitually distracted can be made to become one that is habitually one-pointed or concentrated, by practicing different aspects of meditation. The yogis used the term *samyama* (total control of the mind) to describe this phenomenon.

According to yogis, the entire universe, of which each one of us appear to be a part, is imbibed with the three basic constituents of nature—satwa, rajas, and tamas. Satwa, at the mental level, manifests as clarity and peace; rajas, as fickleness and pain; and tamas, as dullness and depression. All the asana and pranayama practice are evolved by yogis to reduce the effects of rajas and tamas so that the mental space is dominated by satwa. Once satwa takes over the mind's space, such a person becomes fit to meditate or do samyama.

Samyama itself is considered to be made up of three stages. The first stage of meditation, *dharana*, is to remain focused on an object for contemplation—a sublime, uplifting object, such as one's personal deity. You repeatedly attempt to keep the mind focused on the same object even as the mind lapses repeatedly into a state of distraction. Over a period of time, you can keep your mind focused on the object almost continually throughout the entire period of meditation. This stage is referred to as *dhyana* (meditation) and *ekagrata* (one-pointedness). When you remain in this stage and continue with the practice, then one day the mind's space will be fully taken up by the object of contemplation and, in the process, you forget even yourself. The great seers, such as Patanjali, refer to this next stage as *samadhi*. So meditation is a gradual patient process for a mind that is made satwic by prior practices of asanas and breathing exercises.

The objects meditated upon vary. The bar is repeatedly raised to focus attention from gross objects to subtler and subtler objects and thoughts. What are the results? Knowledge—complete knowledge of the objects meditated upon. It is called *sampragna* (total, unambiguous understanding). What is the limit to such knowledge? It is knowing the true nature of oneself. What should be called "I" is the question to which the yogi gets an answer. "But I know who I am; I do not need yoga," you may say; however, the yogis say that the common understanding of what constitutes oneself is erroneous. It requires deep meditation to get the true answer to that question directly.

❧ CHANTING AND MANTRA ❧

DAVID: What is the meaning of the word "mantra"? (see *Yoga for the Three Stages of Life*, chapter 5, Mantrayoga).

RAMASWAMI: The word *mantra* is derived from two roots:

man, which means "to think," and *tra*, "to support/protect." Thus a mantra is literally a sound or word that protects the thinker/mediator. Does the sound have a meaning? Can any sound or word be called a mantra? Can I create a sound and call it a mantra?

A mantra usually refers to a word or sound attributed to a deity, which has no form, but the sound itself is its body. So such deities are called *videhas* or *asariris* (without bodies). And the mantra is discovered after deep penance by a *rishi* (sage). That is why rishis are also known as *manra-darsis* (seers of mantras). So we have the Gayatri mantra, which is said to have been discovered by a sage called Visvamitra; and the deity represented by the mantra is the ultimate reality Brahman, the manifestation of which is considered to be the Sun.

So I cannot create a mantra unless I can know for sure that word represents the deity, in which case the sound can be called a mantra. Else it will have no effect. Furthermore, the word *mantra* has also come to mean prayers and hymns in praise of various deities in the Vedas. A large portion of the Vedas consist of these hymns and prayers and so they too are known as mantras. These mantras normally have a meter, a deity they represent, and a sage who saw the mantra in his/her mind's eye. So when a *sadhaka* (worshipper) uses the mantra in his/her *japa* (repetitive uttering), he/she will acknowledge the meter of the mantra, the deity represented by it, and the sage who discovered it. So when one starts japa of the Gayatri, the fingers are placed on one's head and the sage Visvamitra's name is mentioned; then the fingers are placed on the tip of the nose and the name of the meter, Gayatri, is mentioned and finally the fingers are placed on the heart and the name of the deity, Savita (Sun), is mentioned. Another portion of the Vedas uses these mantras and prescribes rules and procedures to propitiate the deities. This ritualistic portion is known as Brahmanas.

There are mantras not belonging to the Vedas, which are variously known as *laukika mantras*. These are contained in various other works like the *puranas* (myths), *ithihasas* (epics), and other ancient works. A set of twelve names is called *dwadasa mantras*, as we find in the popular Sun salutation. There are 108 mantras of different deities, such as Ganesha, Siva, Vishnu, and Kali, which are known as *ashtottara-sata sankhya mantras*. Then we have very popular 1,008 mantras of different deities like Ganesha, Vishnu, and Siva, which are also used for worship. These are normally taken from the puranas and are known as *sahsra namas*.

Several laukika mantras are also very popular—one of which is the mantra on Rama (an incarnation of Vishnu). The Rama mantra is also known as *tarka mantra* (the mantra that helps one to sail through life without difficulties). *Taraka* here means "boat." Like a boat, the mantra protects the subject from not only drowning but helps to go across the sea of samsara without difficulties. Sage Valmiki became a great composer and writer of the epic called *Ramayana* after repeating the tarka mantra for a very long time. Mahatma Gandhi also is credited with using Rama mantra for a long time. When struck by an assassin's bullet, it is said, he died saying, "Hey Ram." ("Hey Ram" in Sanskrit is vocative case, meaning "Oh Rama.")

DAVID: What is the purpose of chanting? Why do it? Is it just a pleasant activity? Or, does chanting really produce some profound results? You mention in *Yoga for the Three Stages of Life* that Vedic chanting produces a satwic effect. Is it really so? Does it help to weaken the kleshas?

RAMASWAMI: The purpose of mantra japa is to merge with the deity whose mantra one is chanting. The puranas are full of stories of devotees young and old, chanting the mantra of the favorite deity in very difficult tapas asanas (austerity poses) to acquire a vision of the Lord. Sometimes it is done with a motive—to get a boon—or just for the ecstasy of seeing the Lord in the mind's eye. Basically the mantra japa is done with extreme devotion. Faith is a sine qua non for mantra japa. Chanting does produce a profound effect, even according to the *Yoga Sutras*. Chant the mantra, then follow it up with contemplating on the meaning of the mantra, says Patanjali. In fact, according to Patanjali, the ultimate knowledge of oneself and the complete irrevocable peace mind accrue to such a yogi. That being the case, the weakening of the klesas, and the mind becoming satwic (clear) are sure results.

161

DAVID: Why is accuracy, like hitting the right note, so important in Vedic chanting? Is there more leeway when chanting the *Yoga Sutras*?

RAMASWAMI: The Vedic mantras were memorized and, until a few years back, were never written. Vedas were also known as *srutis*, as they were heard and not read from a book. They used to be chanted and heard by the student, who would repeat the same mantra passages several times a day, over and over again, for several days, until the student would know them by heart. I trust the *swaras* (notes) help in memorizing them. When one would miss a word or make a mistake, it would show because the swaras would not tally—intuitively, one would realize that there was a mistake. One would memorize the number of words and lines, and memory would aid the beginning of each paragraph. It was an ingenious way to memorize the Vedas. The So hitting the correct note was necessary to maintain the even flow of the mantras. My family subscribes to a Vedic rendition called Krishna Yajur Veda (the same as Sri. T. Krishnamacharya's). It consists of over eighty chapters and it takes about forty-five hours to chant them once. There are scholars who would recite the whole Krishna Yajur Veda without missing a syllable or chanting a discordant note.

The sutras, such as the *Yoga Sutras*, are not Vedic mantras. Sutras were written to convey a body of knowledge succinctly, with the minimum number of words. Writing sutras was a great art, and a deep knowledge of Sanskrit was required. They were not set to notes as the Vedic mantras were, but in practice the sutras are attempted to be chanted using Vedic notes for convenience, and to break the monotony of prosaic sutra recitation. There are no set rules, and one will find variations in sutra chants by different schools, unlike the Vedic chanting.

DAVID: There are many Vedic mantras, such as Gayatri. What are the yoga mantras? Is the pranava (OM) the only yoga mantra? How do we do japa with this one syllable?

RAMASWAMI: In the *Yoga Sutras of Patanjali*, he mentions pranava as the mantra that represents Isvara. There is no specific mention of other mantras. That does not mean that Patanjali approves of only pranava for use. Elsewhere in the same chapter, he mentions meditating on divinity per one's personal dispositions (*Yeta abhimata dhyanat va*). This would include several deities mentioned in the Vedas. According to Sadasiva, who wrote a commentary on the *Yoga Sutras*, it would mean any orthodox form of worship, which will naturally include several Vedic mantras pertaining to specific deities, such as Siva or Vishnu.

DAVID: Many of the Vedic mantras are supposed to have powers that seem magical. They are said to cure infertility, make dull children smart, bring us wealth and glory, help when we're in litigation, and so on. Do people in this day and age still believe in such things? I would imagine they're regarded as superstition by many.

RAMASWAMI: We must understand that these Vedic mantras were originally written to meet specific desires (*kamya*). In the absence of modern developments, the most important means available at that time was prayer to the superior forces. Even in modern times, there are problems that defy any scientific solution, and many people intuitively turn to God and say an earnest prayer. That faith can cure is a fact, for the faithful. The existence of God, the power of prayer, the existence of heaven and hell, the idea of future births—matters that are beyond the power of reasoning— can neither be proved nor disproved by the nonbeliever. There were people in olden days who did not believe in anything that cannot be scientifically proved or logically convincing like modern times. But there are, again, many people who believe in the efficacy of prayer, even in modern times. When all hopes are gone, prayer and faith could prove to be formidable positive influences.

163

DAVID: With respect to our yoga practice, when is the proper time for chanting? Should the chanting come before or after our practice? Or can it be done anytime? How does it relate to japa and meditation?

RAMASWAMI: My guru, Sri. T. Krishnamacharya, would start every class with an appropriate prayer and end with another. Additionally, if one wants to do chanting or japa and meditation, it may be good to do it after asana and pranayama practice. If the chanting consists of passages, as in Vedic suryanamaskara mantras or the sahasranama (1,008 names of a personal deity in the forms of slokas) or if the chanting is *parayana* (recitation of very long passages) then it can be done separately. Usually these chants are best done in the morning but certain chants can be done at different times, as prescribed.

DAVID: If we are not Hindus and come from another religious tradition, should we be chanting in Sanskrit? I was raised in the Jewish tradition and find it more comfortable to chant in Hebrew. Is there something special about Sanskrit?

RAMASWAMI: There is a long ongoing debate about use of Sanskrit mantras vis-à-vis prayers and chants from other Indian languages, such as Tamil. In many Hindu temples, the temple procedure requires the various procedures be done with Sanskrit mantras, but now several temples have changed to mantras in Tamil or other languages. There is a strong claim that Sanskrit mantras have an inherent effect that may not be available in other Indian languages. It is debatable. Sanskrit, as the name indicates, is a said to be a complete, or perfect, language (*samskita* = "perfectly done").

164

I think if a person has strong religious disposition, it is best to stick to one's own religious practices, as switching to different religious practices could create considerable conflict. In fact Lord Krishna says in the Gita that one should not create religious confusion in others (*na buddhi bhedam janayeth*). Though he refers to intrareligious practices, this could very well apply to interreligious matters. But if a person has no religious moorings, then if he/she likes other chants, such as the Sanskrit chants or prayers or hymns, he/she may take advantage of it. (I also find that many people who have no devotional fervor soon desert these practices.)

DAVID: Is there a difference between chanting in groups and chanting by oneself? Between chanting aloud and chanting silently?

RAMASWAMI: Usually, mantras meant for recitation (parayana) are said aloud, whereas mantras in japa are best done silently. In fact, the japa should be done without even the movement of the lips. The parayana mantras can be chanted aloud individually or in groups. My guru once said that he and a group of some Vedic scholars would go around the streets of Mysore chanting the Sun salutation mantras aloud, so that those who are ill and confined to their homes could listen to at least a few of the mantras that would bring good health and solace to the sick. There is also a very popular chant of Siva from the Vedas known as Rudram (I have included this chant on the CD that accompanies my recent book, *The Complete Book of Vinyasa Yoga*). These are chanted on specific days of the week and special occasions. One such occasion is called

Siva Ratri, the "night of Siva." On Siva Ratri, several people chant the Rudram chant over and over again all over the day and night without a wink of sleep.

Sometimes a great Rudram chant is organized; on such an occasion, offerings are made to Siva with the accompaniment of Rudram chanting, or what is popularly known as Rudra parayana. It is a custom for groups of eleven chanters sitting in a circle and chanting the Rudram, which itself has eleven paragraphs in one voice. In a huge gathering, there may be eleven such groups, each group independently chanting the Rudram in one go. Then each group will repeat the same procedures eleven times all through the day. Then the procedures will be repeated for eleven days all in a public place. Devotees who cannot chant themselves sit and listen to the chants. Hordes of people come and sit for as long as they can and as many times as they can. This procedure is done for the public good, as the mantras are believed to produce auspiciousness to the whole community.

Japa basically is repetition of a mantra that is usually short. Repeating OM several times mentally, as recommended by Patanjali, is called *pranava japa*. Gayatri is another mantra that is repeatedly meditated upon over and over again, three times a day. There are people who chant the Gayatri about a thousand times a day and aim to complete 10 million repetitions in their lifetime.

A mantra gives benefit, it is believed, by more and more repetitions (*aavritti*). The successful use of the mantra is as much in the hands of the mediator as with the mantra itself. The meditator reaps the benefit of his/her own input. Hence careless use, and changing the mantras often, are reasons why many find the mantras unproductive.

DAVID: Were you ever taught to chant during asana? I know there is chanting with suryanamaskara. Is this the only case? What is the difference in effect between suryanamaskara with and without chanting? Might chanting during asana be useful for lengthening the exhale or focusing the mind?

RAMASWAMI: Generally, chanting is done while seated usually in sukhasana, but my teacher used to ask us to sit in various seated yogic poses, such as like vajrasana and padmasana, while chanting or doing Veda parayana. In a sequence called *dingnamaskara* (salutation to the directions), the ding-namaskara mantras are used. Usually, Vedic chanting can be attempted to improve the breathing and also to help the mind focus. Chanting is beneficial to both the mind and breath, and also for the body if done in a proper yogic pose.

DAVID: Can chanting be taught to someone who is tone deaf and can't sing?

RAMASWAMI: I do not know. I have never attempted it.

DAVID: What does *bijaksara* mean? What is a bijaksara mantra?

RAMASWAMI: *Bija* means "seed" and *akshara* is "a letter," or literally "irreducible." Normally, a bija akshara is taken and nasal sound "M" is added to get the bijakshara mantra. There are several theories about the efficacy of these mantras, where in the body they emanate from and the deity associated with the mantras. This particular subject known as *mantra sastra* is quite popular with certain sections of the people. OM, the most revered mantra, is a bijakshara mantra. Hrim is another well-known mantra associated with sakthi (power).

OM

DAVID: In the Mandukya Upanishad (Upanishad of the Atharva Veda), verse 8, it says, "*so'yam atmadhyaksaram aumkaro'dhimatra*"

(This is the self, which is of the nature of the syllable OM, in regard to its elements). What does this mean? How is our true self, the atman, like this sound, OM?

RAMASWAMI: OM is the most sacred Vedic word. It is a one-syllable mantra. Every mantra is integral with a deity, and here the Upanishad uses the mantra OM with paramatma (the Supreme Self), also known as Brahman (that which manifests as the universe). The first seven mantras of the Mandukya Upanishad describe the Brahman in its three aspects, discernable as the waking, dream, and deep-sleep states, and finally the unmanifest state called the *turiya* (fourth).

In this mantra, or passage, referred to in the question, for the sake of meditation, Brahman is related to the mantra OM. The syllable OM, like the Brahman described, has four aspects or elements: A, U, and M, and the whole mantra in an unmanifest state. Each element of the word OM is now identified with one of the four states of consciousness. This is a method of meditating on the Brahman, by using the mantra of Brahman, which is OM.

As we have seen in the *Yoga Sutras*, pranava should be chanted with the *bhavana* (feeling) of the import of the mantra (YS I, 28). That is, when one meditates upon Brahman using the mantra OM, one will associate A with the waking state, U with the dream state, M with the deep sleep state, and the whole mantra with the unmanifest turiya. The way to use a mantra is to make it virtually indistinguishable from the *artha* (the meaning of the mantra). The artha here is the Brahman. Hence, when someone uses the mantra, he/she will consider the mantra to be the Brahman, and meditate as mentioned in the Upanishad. It is said that the mantra sound is itself the body of the deity and hence inseparable from the deity indicated. So the self, or Brahman, is said to be the nature (essence) of OM, having the same number of elements or aspects as the mantra itself. The use of sound, image, or idea is resorted to for the purpose of knowing the Brahman, which is obscure for the ordinary mind. The mind is slowly led to the unknown from the known.

❦ GAYATRI ❧

DAVID: Why do such mantras as the Gayatri require initiation? This sounds like some kind of magical process. Why can't we just learn the mantra (correctly) and use it?

RAMASWAMI: I do not know of anyone in India who does recitation of Gayatri mantra on a regular basis without being properly initiated. It is the belief that any mantra learned without proper initiation (*mantra diksha*) will be ineffective in giving the intended benefit. A student is usually initiated into these mantras (especially Gayatri) at a very young age, by a person who himself has chanted the mantra correctly several thousands of times over a long period of time. There are well-laid-out procedures for mantra chant (japa vidhana). Knowing the correct pronunciation, its import, and proper preparation, like asana and pranayama, are all required to chant the mantra correctly, and all these are covered in the initiation. The recipient of the mantra should emotionally vibrate with the mantra to obtain the intended benefit.

The initiation to the Gayatri mantra is usually done at the time of initiation into Vedic studies (*upanayana*), which enables one to become "twice born" (*dwija*). Because Gayatri is believed to be the essence of the Vedas, considerable importance is given to the proper chanting, knowing the meaning, and doing all the accompanying rituals. Thereafter Gayatri japa is performed daily at dawn, noon, and dusk as part of the worship of the Sun. There are millions of people who have been initiated into Gayatri alone, and to no other mantra, and they become dedicated worshippers of Gayatri. Mantras such as Gayatri are believed to have special vibrations, and an *upasaka* (worshipper) will soon become one with the mantra.

I was initiated into the study of the Vedas at the age of nine, when I was also initiated to Gayatri mantra. As I mentioned, a mantra should be learned from one who has himself attained siddhi (perfection) in the mantra. Since such people are few and far between, it is the custom in India for the father to initiate the child into Vedic studies and the Gayatri. Proper initiation ensures that the student will be quite serious about the practice of the mantra during his/her lifetime and obtain the siddhi. Mantra chants can lead to *saphala* (success), *nishphala* (failure), or *viparita phala* (undesirable results), depending upon various factors. Hence, people in India are very careful about (a) choosing the mantra, (b) choosing the initiator, and (c) choosing additional mantras while not doing enough justice to the mantra already initiated into.

Orthodox belief is that the Vedic mantras, like the Gayatri, were "discovered" by rishis. A rishi is one who sees the mantra in his/her mind's eye after intense tapas (penance). Because he/she has invested considerable mental energy in this discovery (a mantra is not an invention like a poem), he/she is privy to the import of the mantra as well. In ancient times, the scripts were not there, so the mantra was transmitted only to those who were willing to learn and practice, and those who the seer thought fit to use the mantra. He did not merely speak the mantra, but also explained the form of the *devata* (divine being) and the proper use (*prayoga*) of the mantra. All this certainly requires someone to spend time and effort to teach a student who is willing to use it, meditate on it, and repeat it many times. So learning a mantra from a book or from one who him/herself has not attained a semblance of siddhi from sufficient number of repetitions (*aavritti*) is considered inappropriate.

The various sages discovered many mantras. Later on, such sages as Vyasa compiled them into the Vedas, which contain innumerable mantras. These mantras can be chanted or used in rituals for obtaining the necessary boons from the deities associated with the mantras.

Every Vedic mantra has a meter, a seer, and a deity. Thus, in formal chanting of the mantras several preliminaries such as paying respect to the seer, the devata, and the meter itself are done.

Chanting the mantras without knowing the meaning does not yield any results. In the *Yoga Sutras of Patanjali*, referring to Isvara japa, clearly says that the repetition of the mantra should be followed by meditation on the import of the mantra (YS I, 28). That being the case, how can any one know the correct japa of a mantra without instruction from one who has, himself, attained perfection in the mantra? So the use of an initiator is not just desirable but necessary.

DAVID: In YY VI, 11–15 and 16–23: Here Yajnavalkya seems to distinguish between those initiated into the Vedas (Brahmins) and others who haven't been. When it comes to mantra, Brahmins should say Gayatri; women and others, a *namah* (not mine) mantra. Does this mean I should not use Gayatri for pranayama?

RAMASWAMI: I was "baptized," or initiated, into the Vedic way of life, after an elaborate ceremony called upanayana, when I was ten years old. Some children get initiated when they are five or seven years old. One of the important aspects of this initiation ceremony is the teaching of the sacred Vedas to the subject. One mantra from the Vedas is taken and muttered into the right ear of the subject, usually by the father, while both are huddled under the cover of a silk cloth. The mantra is Gayatri mantra, and with that the subject is given permission to study the Vedas. Gayatri mantra thereafter becomes part of the religious life of the subject. The subject, among other things, is required to do *sandhyavandana* (prayer ritual to the Sun) three times a day: at dawn, midday, and dusk. It contains both Vedic and nonVedic prayers and rituals, but essentially requires the subject to do samantraka pranayama about ten times followed by japa of the Gayatri mantra several times. Thus, Gayatri japa becomes the centerpiece of the religious/ spiritual life of all those who have been initiated by upanayana.

Should only Brahmins study the Vedas and hence Gayatri, which is part of Vedas? When I was young, the general belief was that Vedas were to be chanted and the Vedic rites performed only by Brahmins. In fact, Gayatri is seldom chanted aloud; rather, it is said silently so that even the womenfolk in the households will not hear it. The surynamaskara mantra (known as *arunam*), which is part of the Vedas and takes about an hour to recite, contains the Gayatri mantra. When we would come to that while chanting suryanamaskara, we used to say it in a low voice, or even silently, if people were around, lest they hear it. Later on I learned from my teacher that Vedic studies should be done by the three *varnas* (castes): Brahmins (Vedic scholars), Kshatriyas (warriors), and Vaisyas (traders), as you can see from the slokas you have referred to in this question. Actually several smritis mention that, with respect to Vedas, the Brahmin could chant, teach, do Vedic rites or act as a priest for someone else to do the Vedic rites, give gifts for helping the Vedic rites, and receive fees/gifts for teaching the Vedas. However, the other two castes can learn the chants, do the Vedic rites, and give fees for getting religious rites done, but not do the other three functions.

171

There are several commentaries written about the meaning of Gayatri, but basically it is a fervent prayer to the Lord, whose manifestation is considered to be the bright orb of the Sun, to stoke the fire of intellect to realize the spiritual truth. The prayer by itself appears nonsectarian. But was the restriction on Vedic studies brought about at a later date?

Among all rituals, those who study the Vedas consider the initiation rituals of upanayanam to be the most important. In the ancient times, upanayanam is said to have been available to both men and women, of all communities, desiring to study the Vedas. Some of the Brahma *gnanis* (sages), such as Parasara, Vyasa, Sathyakama, and Padmapada, were not born in the high castes, but organized the Vedas and compiled all the karmas for the upanayanam. Even Sage Visvamitra, who is the seer of the Gayatri mantra, was not a Brahmin. In Brahad-Arnyaka Upanishad, Yagnyavalkya teaches the important Brahma vidya to his wife Katyayani. Several scholars mentioned in the Vedas were not Brahmins, and there are Upanishadic stories in which Brahmins went to non-Brahmins to study some aspect of philosophy, even about Brahman. The transformation to a future birth and their contributions are contained in the Vedas. Several scholars and historians say that as the traditions changed after the eighth century AD, it was restricted to persons born into families of the upper classes only, and was denied to women.

In India, among Hindus, the number of Brahmins who study or do the Vedic rituals has dropped dramatically during the last several decades. Many Brahmins have their initiation ceremony but thereafter never perform the daily ritual, sandhyavandana, which requires the subject to chant Gayatri three times each day. For every hundred Brahmins who are initiated, perhaps five do the daily rituals (making a mockery of the initiation ceremony). And out of these five, maybe one will study the Vedas. Some of the old Upanishads refer to such Brahmins as Brahmabandhu (relative of a Brahmin) and not a Brahmin. My guru, Sri. T. Krishnamacharya, I thought, was rather exercised about it and started teaching Vedic chanting to interested women, lest the study of Vedas would become obsolete. Some of his female students chant them beautifully now.

There is a mismatch now. Study and observance of Vedas has been dropping among Brahmins and other Hindus, but interest in these studies is growing among non-Hindu intellectuals. Several of the Western scholars, Max Muller and others, have done great service to the study of Vedas, but on a more intellectual plane. During the last decade, study of Vedic mantras has become popular among non-Hindus, especially the yoga-practicing community. However, these mantras have great potency, and in the initiation and chanting, bhavana becomes necessary. This is lacking. Any carelessness in chanting or in devotion would mean harming or showing disrespect to the deity the mantra relates, and could lead to undesirable consequences to the subject who chants the mantra—such is the conventional belief. On the other hand, I feel that anyone can take to mantra japa, including Gayatri, if he/she would emote with the deity represented by the mantra.

173

The Vedic mantra associated with pranayama is given in my book (*Yoga for the Three Stages of Life*, page 202). There are several pranayama mantras mentioned by several sages (in addition to Yagnyavalkya) in smritis (texts), written by them. For a more detailed treatment of the samantraka pranayama, refer to YTSL, pages 199–206.

ఆ DHYANA ఆ

DAVID: (YR I, 20) Can we practice dhyana? Or is this, again, something the may or may not happen after practice? Is mantra japa a way to practice meditation? We may repeat the mantra, but whether the mind quiets down and stays focused on the mantra, isn't this a siddhi, something we can't control?

RAMASWAMI: Dhyana, or what is translated as "meditation," is, according to Patanjali, an aspect of antaranga sadhana (internal practice). So it is to be considered a practice. *Dhyana* comes from the root word *dhyai*, "to think deeply." The word *dhyana* is not used for all involved thinking. It is used to signify deep thinking of a sublime object, that meditation which will uplift the practitioner. According to my guru and several experts on Bhakti yoga (yoga of devotion), the word *dhyana* can be used only with respect to thinking of the Lord, when it is also known as *Bhagavat dhyana*. In fact, some of the Bhakti yogis do not at all recognize the higher stage of yoga, samadhi. They would say that the ultimate goal of the individual is to be in dhyana of the Lord until death. Deep or obsessive thinking of wordly objects or actions will normally be considered chinta, and not dhyana.

Does it happen to ordinary people? Mostly not, but the causes of that nonaccomplishment are dealt with clearly by yoga texts. If one can work it out correctly, dhyana practice and accomplishments are possible. The mind, or chitta, being an aspect of prakriti, is also made up of the three gunas: satwa, rajas, and tamas. Yogic dhyana is not possible until the mind becomes satwic. This is where many people find they are not able to do dhyana, basically because their minds are predominantly rajasic or tamasic. In the Gita, also, the Lord says that if you are tamasic, become rajasic; if you are rajasic, become satwic; and if you are satwic, go beyond the three gunas (*nistrigunya*). He does not give the procedures to be adopted to achieve this. But yoga sadhana clearly tells us how to proceed.

Basically our chitta is nothing but the remainder of our samskaras, our past actions/habits: *Samskara sesham hi chittam.* So, unless the individual takes steps to replace the old, bad samskaras with newer, wholesome samskaras, he/she will continue to operate on the path driven by the old samskaras. Yoga is the process or practice by which this transformation (*parinama*) is achieved. Since there are individuals and individuals, the set of practices that one can do may not work for another because he/she may not be fit for that kind of practice. For instance, if a person is tamasic, he/she tends to be disorderly, ignorant, sense-pleasure oriented (*aviraga*), and usually is slavish. Most people fall into this category. Rajasic people tend to be fickle-minded, power hungry, possessive, and uneven tempered. Satwic ones are orderly (in their thinking and actions), knowledge oriented, and discriminative (especially between self and nonself), and become moral and spiritual leaders of mankind. People fall into these

reducing the tamas and rajas (that is, without doing the asana and pranayama preliminaries), then during the time of dhyana, the mind either wanders because of rajas or goes to sleep because of tamas (and some mistake those petite episodes of sleep as trance).

Dhyana is therefore the effort to keep the mind focused on one object to the exclusion of all others, during the time period. As this requires practice, one starts with a mantra or an icon or a point inside the body. The first step is to repeatedly bring the mind to the object every time the mind wanders because of the previous samskaras. Here, some willpower is needed, but you are not forcing your mind. You have only to coax the mind back to your object every time you realize that your mind has gone off it. This aspect is called *dharana*, the anga (part) before dhyana or that leads to dhyana. Every time someone mediatates with a mantra, at the end of the meditation, he/she should review the meditation practice: Did my mind wander too often? Was the time duration of my wayward mental activity predominant? With time, the mind will be with the object for a longer span of concentration and the frequency of the distracted state will go down. Then the practitioner knows that he/she is making progress. There may be day-to-day variations. But what is to be seen is whether the quality of dharana is improving. Eventually, the practitioner will be with the object almost the entire duration of the meditation session. Then he/she can conclude that he/she has achieved dhyana. So dhayana is the result of dharana practice. Furthermore, the advice of Patanjali in japa is very important. He says that the mantra japa should be as follows: First chant the mantra and immediately think of the meaning or import of the mantra. Chant the mantra again and then think of the import (*Tat japah tadarthabhavanam*). In this manner, the involvement of the meditator with the mantra is more intense and the chances of the mind wandering are less. Unfortunately, many people chant the mantras mechanically.

When you continue with dhyana practice, the intensity of concentration improves, and you reach the stage where only the object alone is remembered. You even forget yourself in the object, which is the state of samadhi. In essence, dhyana, preceded by dharana and followed by samadhi, is a continuous practice, resulting in the transformation of the mind. Born yogis do not need the preliminaries, but most do.

✌ PRACTICE FOR MEDITATION ✌

DAVID: A friend writes: I have to teach a class on yoga and meditation. What is your advice for a class emphasizing the meditative process?

RAMASWAMI: I suggest the following agenda for meditation class:

1. Begin with a short prayer.
2. Do a tadasan group: Choose about sixteen vinyasas. Do each vinyasa about three times and rest at the end. It may take about 10 minutes.
3. Do vajrasana or paschimatanasana vinyasas and rest at the end. It may take about 8 to 10 minutes for this.
4. Do kapalabhati 108 times (36 times in each of the three positions of the hands).
5. Do ujjayi pranayama sixteen times using the ratio 5:5:10:5 with the bandhas in bhaya kumbhaka (about 10 minutes).
6. Do shanmukhi mudra for 5 minutes.
7. Do trataka (external gazing at a picture of sunrise or flame of a candle or an oil lamp) for 5 minutes. Gaze until the eyes start watering, and then close the eyes. Repeat for a total duration of 5 minutes.

8. Meditate on rising sun or flame. Image the object between the eyebrows or in the heart region. Then image the light dispelling the darkness/depression from the heart or the mind—imagine the light dispelling the darkness or depression like the dew disappearing in the morning with sunrise. Do this alternately for 5 minutes. Open the eyes and review the quality of the meditation. How often the mind wandered from the object of meditation, how long were the distractions? Repeat the exercise for the reminder of the time.

9. At the end, have a short review. Ask a few students to describe the quality of their meditation. Ask them to follow the routine for four weeks. They may change the asana routine, but the other aspects of the regimen may remain the same.

10. End the class with a short prayer.

I hope these ideas are useful. (For the asanas and pranayama, you may refer to *The Complete Book of Vinyasa Yoga* and *Yoga for the Three Stages of Life*.)

❧ OBJECTS FOR MEDITATION ❧

Jyotismati

DAVID: As we acquire deeper and deeper habits of ahimsa (nonviolence) and santosha (contentment), anger will diminish. Let me ask about another approach. I often think of anger and hatred and similar things as a kind of darkness in the heart. In YS I, 36, one of the suggestions Patanjali offers for dealing with an unsteady mind is *jyotismati*, meditation on a radiant light. So, I wonder if this could be helpful: to meditate on the Sun in the heart, a bright, radiant light in our heart, as a way of dispelling the darkness and reducing our anger.

RAMASWAMI: Yes, meditating in the heart with a bright object like the sun is recommended in the Vedas. I have dealt with this subject in some detail in my book *Yoga for the Three Stages of Life*, pages 58–59. But again, the question is: how well can a person meditate when his/her mind is distracted? (Please refer to my answer to the question on dhyana.) Again, the jyotishmati vritti practice is mentioned in the first chapter, which is for the highest *adhikarai* (fit person). So unless one is basically highly satwic, this meditation may not work or may not be possible to do as the mind will always be wandering or showing signs of tamas. So in the scheme of things, we should say that the ability to do any high degree of meditation such as the jyotishmati has a prerequisite of reduced rajas and tamas. This can be achieved by the yama, niyamas, asana, and pranayama, as I have explained in an earlier answer. If a person is predominantly satwic, then he/she can do jyotishmati visualization easily, and possibly he/she need not practice yama niyamas, as he/she was probably born as an *ahimsaite*, possessing all the other traits as well. I would say for the general populace, yama niyama comes first; and then, adding asana and pranayama will enable a yogi to successfully meditate and visualize.

179

DAVID: Am I using the word *meditate* correctly? Would it be more correct to say the *bhavana* (visualization) of bringing the sun into the heart?

RAMASWAMI: Yes, bhavana will be a better term for abstract-object meditation. In fact, my guru would say, "Image the rising sun between eyebrows" (the area known as *bhrumadhya*). He would use the English word "imagine."

Breath

DAVID: Is the breath considered an uplifting object to focus on?

RAMASWAMI: Yes, sir.

Patanjali's Suggestions

DAVID: You've mentioned a few times that chapter I of the *Yoga Sutras* is meant for the more advanced yogi, the one who is already capable of samadhi, a focused and steady mind. Does this mean (as in your answer on jyotismati) that the suggestions Patanjali gives for steadying an unsteady mind (YS I, 32–39) are really not of much practical use for the average or beginning yoga student?

RAMASWAMI: Since we seem to be coming back to this question, let us try another approach. One who wants to meditate but does not care for all the preliminaries should start doing meditation of jyotis in one's heart or middle of the eyebrows, focusing on the light principle for, say, 15 minutes, both morning and evening, for four weeks. As I mention in my answer to the question on dhyana, one should review one's experience of meditation periodically. At the end of this four-week exercise, one should look back on the experience to see if the quality of one's meditation has improved. Is one's attention span greater? Are the distractions fewer? Does one feel refreshed at the end of the meditation? Or fall asleep during meditation? Do other thoughts intervene at regular intervals? If it is yes, and emphatic yes for an answer, then this meditation is really good for the person. If there are no improvements, if the student becomes less and less enthusiastic about the practice, if the student forces him/herself to do this in the hope that somehow it will work in the course of time, as if by a miracle, then perhaps he/she can conclude that he/she still has to prepare himself before practicing meditation.

In the preamble to his commentary to the second chapter of YS, Sadhana Pada (the chapter on practice), Vyasa is quite clear in helping to demarcate the levels of yoga. He says, "The yoga attained by a yogi with engrossed mind (samahita chitta) has been stated. This sutra (the first of the second chapter) starts to indicate how a devotee (yogabhyasi) with a restless mind can also attain yoga."

So it is a question of whether the beginner or average yogi has the capability to be engrossed—samahita chitta is the characteristic of the yogi of the highest order, described in the first chapter. For such a yogi the means are *abhyasa* (practice) and *vairagya* (dispassion). The yogi who has the capability to remain engrossed in an object transforms himself into a yogi whose mind is completely in a state of nirodha. This presupposes that unless a yogi has the capability to be completely in samadhi, he/she will not be able to progress to the level of kaivalya attained by vairagya practice. Such a yogi, even as he/she practices to transform his/her mind, may occasionally slip into a state of distraction due to some remaining past karmas or carelessness. To prevent such slippage developing into a fall, the first chapter suggests a few well established yoga practices in YS I, 32–39, as you mention. It is virtually a safety net. In this is included the jyotishmati practice as well. Obviously, a beginner-level practitioner will not be able to practice correctly and successfully. Conversely, if a beginning student is able to successfully practice these yoga meditations, one can conclude that he/she is actually a high-level yogi fit for samadhi yoga as described in the first chapter.

Others should go through the sadhana detailed in the second chapter. Then they will see that, after all these external (*bahiranga*) practices, the yoga practitioner is able to be more focused, practice dharana and dhyana, and then achieve samadhi. These are again described in the third chapter.

You will see that the same jyotishmati practice mentioned as a corrective device in the first chapter is described as a siddhi in the third chapter. In YS III, 31, it is said that by doing samyama or jyotishi in the middle of the eyebrows, the yogi is able to see the *siddhas* (those who have attained extraordinary achievements).

181

Similarly samyama in *hradaya* (heart) (YS III, 33) will lead to understanding one's own mind. Likewise other practices mentioned in YS I, 32; *maitri karuna* (friendliness, compassion) and others mentioned as practices for siddhi in the third chapter, YS III, 23, *Maitriyadisu* (yogic contemplation on friendliness).

So I may summarize by saying that if a yogi does not have the capability to be engrossed or totally focused, then he/she has to do practices that will enable him/her to get the necessary capability. The entire second chapter with all the external practice is to prepare the yoga practitioner to become a yogi.

Dreams

David: In YS I, 38, Patanjali suggests meditating on dreams as one of the methods for making the mind steady. Is this the same as examining dreams in psychotherapy, searching out their meaning, trying to understand them, or is something else being referred to here?

Ramaswami: Some of the contemporary yoga scholars do talk about analyzing the dreams to read one's own mind. I would like to mention what the commentators of years gone by have to say.

In *Yoga Sudhakara*, Sadasiva, writing an independent commentary, says, "By meditating upon such scripturally fascinating substance, as has been seen in dream, and on delight as has been experienced in deep sleep, the mind supported by such objects, becomes steady and obtains the state of one-pointedness." Many authors describe divine vision in the dream (*divyam swapnam*) as appropriate object of repeated reflection. And a restful deep sleep is called satwika nidra. Most people most of the time have dreams which border on being nightmares, and seldom have deep sleep. Actually these two, divine dreams and blissful sleep, are results of a samhita, an engrossed mind.

Freedom or Bondage

DAVID: In YY IX, 1, Yajnavalkya states that dhyana can lead to freedom or bondage. Is this a way of stating the importance of the object we choose for meditation? That if we choose the wrong object, we are led in the wrong direction?

RAMASWAMI: The second half of the sloka which you are referring to is an oft-quoted saying that you find in some other ancient works, with a slight variation. Instead of *dhyana* the word is *manas* (mind), which of course implies the same. So the quote will be, "Mind is the cause of freedom or bondage of beings." Yagnyavalkya's quote will be: "Dhyana [meditation, or literally 'thinking'] is the cause of freedom or bondage of beings."

Dhyana refers to deep, persistent thinking of or about an object, which is meditation. So the idea Yagyavalkya conveys here is that, depending upon what you think, you become either a transmigratory person or a free person. For you to become a free person, he suggests different types of meditation on the ultimate reality, Brahman, which he enumerates in the entire chapter.

My guru used the word *dhyana* for the uplifting meditation, or the meditation on the form of the Lord. He, as a Bhakti yogi, would say, "There is only one dhyana and that is Bhagavat-dhyana (meditation on the Creator)."

Some of us may be obsessed with such things as power, wealth, fame, or sensual pleasures, and think of it all the time. These thoughts are bondage producing, from the viewpoint of the Raja yogi who wants total liberation (kaivalya). So, depending upon what you are obsessed with, depending upon what goes on in the mind all the time, one becomes free or in bondage. My guru used the word *chinta* to indicate obsessive mental focus on worldly or otherworldly accomplishments, such wealth or going to heaven, as the kind of focus leading to bondage.

The word *dhyana*, in this sloka you have referred to, should be considered to mean both meditation and obsession.

Meditating on Isvara

DAVID: In discussing the concept of Isvarapranidhana in chapter I of the *Yoga Sutras*, the suggestion is made that we meditate on Isvara as pure consciousness because this is easier than discovering our self. So, should we choose this as a good first step?

RAMASWAMI: Some teachers, like my guru, assert that this is the only way (*va* = only), but for some others, especially those Samkhya yogis who are not comfortable with the principle of Isvara, the elaborate understanding of the twenty-five principles will be the only way. So for the yogi who can go into samadhi of Isvara, as Isvarapranidhana is mentioned in the context of the first chapter, it could be the best way.

Prana Upasana vs. Mantra Upasana

DAVID: Prana upasana vs. mantra upasana: By focusing on the prana in prana upasana, we are focusing on an object of prakriti (nature). But, since mantra is a link to the Divine, in mantra upasana we are focusing on some aspect of God that does not belong to prakriti. So, would mantra upasana be of a different nature than prana upasana?

RAMASWAMI: If we follow the *Yoga Sutras*, which are said to be Raja yoga (yoga of light), the objective of the whole exercise is to know—to know the nature of all the aspects of prakriti, to know the nature of the unmanifest prakriti (*mula prakriti*), and to know also the true nature of the subtlest principle, which should be called the self. Basically it is knowledge of everything, that the yogi is after. He/she will know all the principles to be known by practicing total yogic concentration. Knowing each and every principle, he/shethen develops disinterest in everything, and finally understands the subtlest principle, which is his/her self; which is nothing but unchanging pure consciousness. Even his/her devotion to Isvara or God (note: God in Patanjala's scheme of things is not the Creator.) is to gain the knowledge of his/her own self through the grace of God.

185

So the yogi is after the capacity to concentrate, or samyama. To get this capability, he/she does the bahirangas, the external practices, before he/she becomes fit to start the samyamas on an object. Now the object, to start with, can be prana; because prana is there to be observed, unlike other objects like an icon or a mantra. Objects like an icon or a mantra have to be connected to initially and periodically brought before the mind.

Once he/she develops the habit of easily going into samadhi on one object, he/she can take other more subtle objects and get into the appropriate *sampragnata* (knowledge-producing samadhi).

The Samkhyas and yogis do not refer to other mantras. The only mantra the yogi refers to is pranava. He/she would like the abhyasi to use this mantra not for the vision of God or material prosperity or otherworldly benefits, but only for the knowledge of the self.

But if you are a Bhakti (devotion) yogi, it is different cup of tea. The Bhakti yogi is after the vision of his/her favorite deity (Ishtadevata), which is represented by the mantra. Even for Bhatki yogis, it will be a good idea to practice observance of the breath, achieve the capacity to concentrate, and then do mantra japa of the favorite deity. Even the formal mantra japa practice traditionally requires the devotee to do a few pranayamas before doing the mantra japa.

DAVID: As regards prana upasana, is the idea to focus on the prana? Or, would we say that the idea is to focus on the breath and that the breath is linked to the prana? Can we say that when we focus on the breath, we are focusing on the prana and vice versa, when we focus on the prana we are focusing on the breath?

RAMASWAMI: Prana is the neurological or the biological force or energy that is responsible for the act of breathing. Due to this force, breathing takes place. The energy giving prana vayu goes in and the waste air comes out. So the prana upasana refers to the observance of this force.

Where is it located? Where does it manifest? It is at a point inside the chest, from where inhalation appears to start and into which exhalation ends. The yogabhyasi carefully focuses his/her attention to that spot and remains observant. It may be done for a few minutes in the beginning of the exercise. Thereafter, even when the abhyasi is doing deep inhalation and exhalation, he/she can do it without the mind wandering away from the pranasthana.

When one practices inhalation and exhalation with the focus in the correct position, there is considerable improvement in the length of both inhalation and exhalation, and one also gets very good control over pranayama.

❧ TRATAKA ❧

DAVID: HYP II, 32 states that the practice of trataka (gazing) overcomes sloth. Why is this so?

RAMASWAMI: Trataka is of two kinds, external and internal. Trataka usually has a light, a flame as the object. Later on, the practitioner attempts to keep the same luminous object in the mind's eye as he/she closes the eyes. It becomes a practice similar to jyotishmati vritti. And light is said to dispel darkness that is tamas. Many people in the initial stages will not be able to visualize light in their heart, but by starting with the external trataka on light, he/she can subsequently do the practice internally.

David: What is antah trataka?

Ramaswami: *Trataka* is "gazing." *Antah* is "inside." You gaze at an object, say, a lamp or candle flame, for a length of time without blinking and until the eyes start watering. This is external gazing. Then close your eyes and "image" the same object with eyes closed. This will be antah trataka.

187

ON THE CHAKRAS

David: In the comment to YR I, 58, it states that if the breathing rate is reduced, that the rotation of the chakras also gets reduced. Why are the chakras spinning? Is the idea that, when the chakras are spinning faster, we are wasting more energy?

Ramaswami: Yes, because the rotation of the chakras (translated as "wheels") is associated with energy level. Yoga tries to reduce the dissipation of energy, and so for the yogi the preference would be having his/her chakras spinning slowly. In fact, the aim of yoga is to reduce excessive metabolic activity. (Excessive metabolic activity could be anger, overindulgence, or other outward-focused preoccupations.) So when one does asanas and pranayama, the metabolic rate as measured by heart rate and, equally important, breath rate comes down.

The breath rate, which is about sixteen per minute, increases during hard work, excessive agitation, anger, and so on. Sustained yoga practice reduces the basal metabolic rate as manifested by lower breath rate. There is an interesting angle to the breath rate. According to one school of Indian philosophers, the lifespan is predetermined. But it is measured in number of breaths. So if you can reduce your breath rate consistently by 10 percent, maybe you would live longer by a few more years.

There is another meaning for the word *chakra*: a collection or a group of certain objects or a cluster of objects. The body consists of a network of nadis (pathways) connected through several nodes, or hubs. Where they are joined in a cluster, that nodal point can be called a chakra. So *chakra* or *nadi-chakra* can mean a node or hub to which or from which several nadis merge or radiate, as if the spokes in a wheel. In which case, the idea of rotation associated with a wheel need not be entertained. In *Hatha Yoga Pradipika*, the commentator translates *nadi-chakra* as *nadi-samuha*, or a family or group of nadis.

188

DAVID: If I think of a chakra as a node connecting nadis, then it's easy to imagine energy flowing through the nadis and through the chakra. But, when I try to think of chakras as spinning wheels, they become more mysterious. The rotation of the chakra is associated with energy level, and, the faster the wheel is spinning, the more energy is being dissipated—but is prana flowing through or around the wheel and somehow causing it to spin? Is the chakra part of the flow of prana, or something the prana flows through? Would you say a bit more on this topic?

RAMASWAMI: According to *Yoga Yagnyavalkya*, when the union of prana and apana is achieved by Hatha yoga practice, the hot prana forces the kundalini to release its obstruction of the sushumna nadi. And through the fine sushumna nadi, the prana moves up, followed by the kundalini. Prana pierces through the six chakras and finally reaches the sahasrara, the ultimate union.

Again, *Hatha Yoga Pradipika*, while talking about the *nadi shodhana* (nadi-cleansing) pranayama, also talks about the inability of the prana to move through the clogged nadis. If you consider nadis and chakras as part of a system, it is appropriate to infer that prana flows through the nadis (and chakras) and not around it. In this regard, considerable visualization is involved.

Once, my teacher mentioned to me that it is not possible to open the body to locate or see the chakras. Perhaps he had just answered the question from a student who wanted to know where exactly in the physical body the chakras are located. He went on to say that the chakras are subtle and cannot be seen, and that the moment you open the body, they get obscured.

He also would mention that the chakras do not rotate with a vertical axis. He would hold his index finger pointing down and rotating it to emphasize that the rotation is not horizontal. I have seen several people say that the main chakras rotate around the three main nadis along the vertical *merudanda* (spine). But, he would say that the chakras rotate with a horizontal axis. He kept his index finger straight, pointing at me, and rotated it like a windmill.

Nadis and chakras are mentioned and discussed in considerable detail in Ayurveda, Hatha yoga, Kundalini yoga, and even Mantra yoga.

The whole approach of yoga is to help the practitioner to turn inward and understand his/her system, be it the body, the nadis, the mind, or the soul. All of these would help to make the yogi less and less interested in the objective universe, and become more and more aware of himself or herself. So it is more a question of an inward journey or study.

Raja yoga urges the yogi to understand his/her's mind and quiet it, so that the mind can see the self forever. Hatha yoga would like the prana that is flowing outward, through the nadis to the senses to experience the external world, to flow inward into the sushumna and reach the sahasrara and obtain samadhi. Kundalini yogis, with some yoga practice and intense visualization, arouse the sleeping kundalini that obstructs the flow of prana to sushumna, and reach the Siva principle, or tatwa, in the sahasrara. This union of sakthi with Siva is the aim of Kundalini yogis, and takes place with intense concentration within the yogi. The same for Mantra yoga. The Sakta Mantra yogis, by intense devotion and use of the mantras, are able to arouse the kundalini and guide it through the sushumna for merger with the Siva tatwa.

189

All these yogas, as you can see, are for the inward journey. All of them promise that, if you are able to reach the goal, the experience is incomparably superior to anything that one gets in this world or the world beyond, like heaven. Kundalini yogis say that, when the ultimate union or yoga is accomplished, the yogi experiences immense bliss throughout his/her nadis. Raja yogis such as Patanjali talk about immense peace in kaivalya. In the *Mahabharata*, a great epic, it is said that the happiness one gets from fulfillment of desires, or the happiness one gets by the fulfillment of the desires in the worlds beyond, such as heaven, is, by comparison, not even a sixteenth part of the happiness one gets out of the desirelessness (vairagya) toward these objects.

DAVID: Also in YR I, 67, it mentions that through the practice of uddiyana bandha (abdominal lock) that chakras become clean and strong. I suppose a chakra's being clean means that energy flows easily, just as with a nadi. And strongly—does this mean the flow of prana will be strong? Or, that the prana will not be dissipated?

RAMASWAMI: Whether you are looking outward for enjoyment of the external world and its myriad objects, or want to traverse the internal journey as the yogi does, the prana should flow freely in either direction. If the nadis and chakras are clogged with impurities, then you become sick and cannot enjoy the worldly life. Nor will you able to make the inward journey, because the yoga (union) of prana and apana and the subsequent inward journey through the sushumna is not possible. So one obtains neither worldly pleasure nor inward happiness if the nadis and chakras are clogged.

My teacher used to compare pranayama to a blower that blows away all the dirt accumulated in the nadis and chakras. He would say that impure nadis cause several diseases, including paralysis, due to the obstructed or weak flow of prana through the chakras and nadis.

DAVID: Are chakras something the beginning or average yoga

student should pay attention to? Can he/she be aware of them? See them? Feel them? Or is that really for the advanced practitioner?

RAMASWAMI: Yes, the chakras can be seen or felt. According to Hatha yogis, the muladhara chakra is located in the *muladhara* (rectal) region. The *svadhishtana* chakra is located in the *lingasthana*, the region of the prostate. Around the navel is *manipuraka*. In the heart region is *anahata*, in the throat is *visudhi*, and between eyebrows is *agna*.

191

Having located the chakras, one goes about accessing them by specific asanas, pranayama, and mudras. By drawing up the rectum, perineum, and glutei (in mula bandha), one is able to access the muladhara. By lifting the pelvic floor (at the beginning of uddiyan bandha), one is able to access the svadhishtana chakra. By drawing in the rectus sheath, one is able to work on the manipuraka chakra. By drawing in the diaphragm, at the end of uddiyana bandha, one is able to access the anahata. By contracting the throat, as in jalandhara bandha, one is able to feel the visuddhi chakra. Sitting in shanmukhi mudra and directing one attention to the middle of the eyebrows, one is able to unite with agna chakra. For the correctness of the bandhas, see the picture of my guru doing all the bandhas on page 81 of *Yoga Rahasya*, 1998 edition.

Mantra yogis and some yogis who practice Kundalini yoga are able to visualize the chakras as the kundalini goes through them one by one. Vivid descriptions of the chakras, in visual terms, are given in many texts. I quote below the experience of H. H. Sankaracharya, of Sringeri Mutt, taken from a book, *Yoga, Enlightenment and Perfection*, containing the teachings and experience of the very highly respected acharya in South India who was the spiritual guru of several communities in India, including our family.

Question: Did Acharya apprehend the chakras?

Answer: Yes. When the sensation arrived at the base of the back, I momentarily beheld the lotus of the muladhara in bloom. Very shortly thereafter, I had a fleeting view of the svad-hishtana. Just before the sensation ascended my back to the level of my navel, I beheld the lotus of the manipura facing downwards, with the petals almost fully closed. The lotus became upright and bloomed when the sensation reached it. Similar was the case with anahata, visuddha and ajna chakras.

One word of caution about these practices is necessary here. This will have to be learned from a much evolved person, spiritually and morally (Sadachara).

❧ HATHA AND RAJA YOGA ❧

DAVID: In Brahmananda's commentary to HYP II, 12, he talks about pratyahara, dharana, dhyana, and samadhi as progressions in pranayama. That is, for instance, when the prana is held (in the Brahmarandhra) for a certain amount of time, it is pratyahara; when it is held there longer, it is dharana. I've never seen these inner limbs of Astanga yoga described this way. Does this amount to the same thing as Patanjali's description?

RAMASWAMI: When I first read *Hatha Yoga Pradipika*, the impression I got was that Svatmarama was usurping the terms of classical yoga and making it appear that his Hatha yoga was complete by itself. In the beginning, he says that his Hatha yoga is like a ladder, a stepping-stone to the more sublime Raja yoga or yoga of Light. Brahmananda, in his commentary, equates the Raja yoga mentioned by Svatmarama to the yoga of Patanjali. Is there a contradiction coming later on?

When Patanjali talks about citta vritti, he talks about nirodha—not of all the functions of the citta, only the thought-vrittis: pramana, and the other four. But citta also has another important function: to maintain life. This, the samkhyas call the *samanya* (karana) vritti—"the general function of the citta." Raja yogis, by completely understanding all the twenty-five tatwas through samadhi (including dhyana and dharana), would bring about the nirodha of the citta, whereas Hatha yogis attempt to stop the functioning of citta through the control of prana. Furthermore, meditation, or more precisely samyama on prana and the absolute withdrawal and control of prana, enables the Hatha yogi to stop the functioning of the citta. The Hatha yogi does not involve himself with other tatwas because prana is an important vritti of citta, and for him/her the control of prana is a necessary and sufficient condition to achieve the goal.

My teacher used to say that one should do pranayama for twice the amount of time one practices asana. Dharana should be for twice that time, and dhyana twice longer. Only then will one be able to stay in samadhi for a fleeting moment. With continuous practice, one will be able to stay in samadhi for longer and longer periods until, like the yogis of Himalaya, one can remain in samadhi for days.

But are the two goals, kaivalya of the Raja yogi and the positioning of prana in Brahmarandhra (a chakra) of the Hatha yogi, the same? Well, one leads to kaivalya or total release and the snapping of the cycle of samsara, but what of the other? One is not sure if the Hatha yogi's goal will give total release from samsara. What do you think?

DAVID: Just to be clear: You are saying that, for Patanjali, nirodha does not mean cessation of all the functions of the mind (for then we would fall down), but only the thought functions? The vrittis that maintain the body functioning remain? And, even in samadhi, where we normally think there is only one vritti, these other (body function) vrittis are still active? Is this the case?

RAMASWAMI: Yes, the yogi continues to live during samadhi, and after he/she gets out of samadhi. Samkhya, the twin philosophy of yoga, gives the example of the potter's wheel to clarify this point. In *Samkhya Karika*, verse 67, Isvarakrishna mentions that even after attaining the ultimate goal of kaivalya, life is maintained by the samskaras of the brain. The yogi continues to eat and breathe, the heart continues to pump blood, and so on. Even after the potter has finished the work and removes the earthen pot from the wheel, the potter's wheel continues to spin for a few more times before it comes to rest. The potter does not stop the wheel, but the wheel stops on its own after the initial momentum given by the potter is used up.

The yogis have tremendous control over the physical, the physiological, and the psychological aspects of themselves. They can control several aspects of their brain functions. They can stop the heart for a while and reduce the breath rate to extremely low levels. But, after they come out of their trance, their siddhi state, their body will function like a normal being (or nearly), even as their mind is in a state of absolute peace (nirodha).

DAVID: But, can't we also say it is the five *prana vayus* (prana, samana, udana, vyana, apana), the five life forces, that are responsible for the functioning of the body? And, probably, when a vayu is active, something corresponding must be active in the brain, some vritti? So, the five vayus controlling the functioning of the body implies a link between the vayus and the samanya (karana) vritti of the Samkhyas.

Furthermore, can we say that the five pranas remain active during samadhi or nirodha?

RAMASWAMI: Yes. Isvarakrishna, the author of Samkhya Karika, agrees with you. The second half of the twenty-ninth sloka says precisely that. The samanya (karana) vrittis are the five vayus. As long as the bodily functions continue, its vayus are also functional.

A detachment with the body and the rest takes place in the

mind of the yogi in kaivalya or the state of nirodha. This can take place in the yogi at any time in the present life—it can take place here and now. Because of the detachment, the activities of the yogi are neither good nor bad, neither merit nor demerit producing, and hence there is no accumulation of karmas.

A similar state is mentioned by the Samkhyas. The Advaita Vedantins also talk about moksha (final release), as occurring during the present life. Such a person is called *jivan mukta*—one who has attained total release *even while living*. It is a state of total detachment. It is a state in which "psychological" death (no attachment, no hatred) takes place before the physiological death.

Several ancient texts, including the Gita, describe the distinguishing marks of such a person. The Buddhist also talks about the state of a liberated person, the one who has attained nirvana, also in a similar vein, I reckon.

This state is, however, contested by other philosophies, especially religion-based philosophies such as Visishtadwaita and, perhaps, by many religions. The devotee/practitioner will continue to do his/her prescribed duties/surrender to the Lord, and the release takes place at the time of death. He/she merges with the Lord or reaches heaven, the Lord's abode. Then there is no rebirth to such a soul. For such a person, there is no total release possible until he/she leaves the body as well.

✾ PRATYAHARA ✾

DAVID: What is the literal meaning of *shanmukhi*?

RAMASWAMI: Shat means "six" and *mukha* means "ports" or "openings." The six ports or holes referred to in shanmukhi mudra are the two eyes, the two ears, the nose, and the mouth. By closing these, we prevent the senses from contacting with the respective objects. It is pratyahara, or one form of pratyahara.

DAVID: I sometimes feel pratyahara is out of order among the eight limbs of Patanjali's Astanga yoga. It's true that when we practice shanmukhi mudra we can successfully close off the senses. But, when we lower our hands and sit quietly, repeating a mantra or focusing on an object, then it is our success at dharana or dhyana that determines whether we can really withdraw prana from the senses. Shouldn't dharana and dhyana come first? And then pratyahara?

RAMASWAMI: We would like to make the mind free of all distractions. Yamas are supposed to reduce the distractions caused by the external world, niyamas to reduce or eliminate the distractions to the mind caused by personal habits. Asanas are expected to make the body healthy—the blood circulation, respiration, digestive systems—everything functions well.

Why does a yogi want a healthy body? Because when he/she wants to contemplate on the distinction between the self and the nonself, which is extremely difficult (again basically because of habit), he/she would like to completely forget the body. The body should not be a source of distraction. The yogi wants a mind free of the woolliness. Pranayama removes the tamas from the mind.

Then the yogi resorts to pratyahara to train the indriyas (senses) to become passive. The senses should also be trained to become quiet. Several pratyahara methods are suggested in the yoga texts, one of which is shanmukhi mudra. In shanmukhi mudra, since the mind still is not trained for meditation, we try to use the breath for the mind to have an anchor.

So all the five external means of yoga—yama, niyama, asana, pranayama, and pratyahara—have a role to play:

Control your relations to the environment (yama).

Control the wrong or nonyogic habits, such as lack of cleanliness, or lack of contentment. Control the karmendriyas (organs of action), such as speech, or the mouth's intake of unwholesome food. Correct the lack of proper yogic knowledge by study. Surrender to the Lord, to remove the nagging burden of all care. All these are achieved by niyama.

Asanas control the body, pranayama clears the mind, and pratyahara specifically targets the senses, which keep on distracting by drawing the yogi toward sensory objects. When all these are taken care of, the mind is then in a fit condition to do dharana and other internal practices. According to Ashtanga yoga, success (siddhi) in all the first angas are necessary conditions before one can really succeed in dharana, etc.

Some born yogis may not need the preliminaries and can go into dhyana or samadhi, but most aspirants need to practice these prerequisites.

DAVID: What are some of the other methods suggested for the practice of pratyahara, besides shanmukhi mudra?

RAMASWAMI: Some old yoga texts, such as Sandilya Upanishad (from the Atharva Veda), talk of different methods of pratyahara, apart from the well-known shanmukhi mudra or yoni mudra.

One other method is to slowly and deliberately withdraw awareness from all the body and direct it inward. In this condition, the yogi is able to withdraw the senses, so that even touching the skin will not create even a ripple in the mind of the yogi. If you lift the yogi's leg, it will drop limp.

This pratyahara is also normally done after pranayama, when the yogabhyasi lies on the floor, with all the joints loose and his/her head tilted to one side, like a dead body. This is known as savasana. In this not only the yogi's pose looks like a dead body, but also, by withdrawing the sensations it will appear to be dead. One draws the sensations slowly and successively from the soles, toes, the heels, knees, groins, rectum, pubis, navel, heart, gullet, palate, nose, and eyes, middle of the eyebrows, forehead, and the crown. One keeps the focus on awareness in the crown, then brings them back in the reverse order. This exercise of withdrawing sensations from the vital/secret positions (*marmasthana*) is another pratyahara.

The Vedantin's perception that everything is atman (self) is another pratyahara. Because one is able to see only the self everywhere and in everything, one has no desire for acquiring anything and hence not distracted by the senses. For the same reason, one dislikes nothing and the senses do not produce any negative feeling toward anything and therefore no object disturbs one.

There are several duties that are obligatory, to be done daily (*nitya*) and ordained to be done at specific times (*vihita*). When one does both but develops a complete disinterest in the benefits arising out of the action, this is another pratyahara—surrender of the results of action. Since, in this way, one has no interest in any object, no object is either desirable or undesirable, the senses will become quiet.

A deliberate attempt to completely avoid (*parang mukhatwam*) contact with objects (as in renouncing them) is still another from of pratyahara.

Some yogis say that all of the forms of pratyahara should be practiced.

DAVID: Is yoni mudra the same as shanmukhi?

RAMASWAMI: My understanding is that they refer to the same procedure. *Shanmukha* refers to the six ports (mukha) in the head/face: the two eyes, the two ears, the nose, and the mouth. Hence is this name given. *Yoni* means "origin" or "orifice." Here, it would mean "the senses," locations through which we take in matter/sensations from the outside world.

5

On Yoga Therapy

INTRODUCTION

YOUGIKA CHIKITSA (YOGA THERAPY) is an approach of using yoga techniques for the treatment of several ailments. The yogi who was after "truth," and thence spiritual freedom, had to find ways and means to be free from ailments so that he could pursue his goal without let or hindrance. By following yama niyamas, he attempted to make complete peace with the external world. Since he sought freedom, he depended upon himself completely to take care of his health needs. He did not want to be dependent upon physicians, surgeons, or a regimen of pills, injections, and Ayurvedic concoctions.

He developed several techniques to promote his own health. He developed several postures and movements called vinyasas, so that he could exercise all the joints, muscles, and tissues. By these asana practices, he ensured that circulation of fluids in the body, such as *raktha* (blood) and *nina* (lymphatic fluids) would move freely. He could access and exercise every joint. Proper nourishment of all the tissues, elimination of waste products, and nourishment of every cell was ensured by the scientific asana and vinyasa practice. Depending upon the specific requirements, he modified the exercise regimen and achieved a healthy system. He also found that his mind was getting more focused, that he was less agitated, and that he felt less and less pain in general, thus becoming more tolerant. The Upanishads marveled at this system of yoga and said that asanas eradicated disease.

200   He made use of the innovative yogic breathing exercises to clear the respiratory system of all the dross, and brought the breathing function more and more under his own voluntary control. By focusing attention on every aspect of breathing: the exhalation, inhalation, and breath-holding—all individually and collectively—he mastered prana, the life force. He ensured that he would never suffer from the debilitating breathing problems. His vital capacity improved, and he could put up with more physical hardships. He also discovered that once he was able to bring his breathing under greater and greater voluntary control, he was also able to have even better control over his own mind. His thoracic spine was strengthened. The deep, slow inhalation also helped to improve the venous return of the blood, thereby helping the heart in its function. Such exercises as kapalabhati (rapid abdominal breathing) also had a direct effect on his heart, as the diaphragm gently massaged it. The deep, conscious, deliberate breathing exercises also had a tonic effect on his nervous system, and thus he could have a better control over his sympathetic and vagus nervous systems. By achieving better control over the sympathetic nervous system, he could control its allergic reactions better. He also found that by the regular breathing exercises, several of the common afflictions of the mind, such as depression, were not to be found in him. He also used the breath-holding time to start focusing attention on different parts of the body or organs or his personal deity, and derived physiological and psychological benefits.

He also theorized that diseases slowly developed due to the displacement of various organs (kosas) inside the body. These internal saclike organs—the heart, the lungs in the thoracic cavity, the stomach, intestines, uterus/prostrate, and bladder—all tended to sag over time due to loss in tone of the supporting musculature. This displacement was, according to him, an important cause of the inefficiency of these important organs. He attempted to correct this situation by resorting to some unique yogic innovations, the *viparita karanis* (inversions). By staying in the inverted position, with asanas such as headstand or shoulder stand and their variations, he found that the organs could be returned to their original position, if practiced for a sufficient amount of time daily. Additionally he used the bandhas (locks) such as mula bandha and uddiyana bandha, to access and massage the various pelvic organs. He found that by these exercises he could access and massage and manipulate any organ—almost—in the body, and keep them in good shape.

He also made use of the power of meditation, to keep the mind under check. He directed the mental energy to sublime thoughts and spiritual matters, and thereby maintained a very healthy mind. With a strong, pure mind in a healthy body, he marched toward the fulfilling goal of spiritual freedom.

⁂ CHIKITSA TEXTS ⁂

DAVID: In regard to the study of chikitsa krama (yoga therapy), you mention the study of several old yoga texts. What are these? Are they the same as the texts you mention in *Yoga for the Three Stages of Life*, chapter 15?

RAMASWAMI: Yes. My teacher had referred to some of these texts and more, such as *Rajayoga Ratnakaram, Hathayogapradipika, Yoga Taravali* (a work on yoga by Sankara), *Yoga Phala Pradipika, Ravana Nadi, Bhairava Kalpam, Sri Tatwanidhi, Yoga (Ratna) Kurantam* (a yoga text written by Kuranta), *Manu Narayaneeyam,*

Rudrayamilam, Brahmayamilam, Atharvana Rahasyam, Patanjala Yoga Darsana, Ghernda Samhita (a Hatha yoga text), *Kapila Sutra* (a Samkhya text), *Yoga Yagnyavalkya, Siva Samhita* (a Hatha yoga text), *Narada Panchratra Samhita* (text on Vaishnavite ritual), *Suta Samhita, Sambhu Rahsya,* and several Upanishads I had mentioned in my book, including Dhyana Bindu, Sandilya, Yoga Sikha, Yoga Kundalini, Nadabindu, Amritabindu, and Garbha. He had also researched several unpublished palm leaf manuscripts. He once exhorted us (the lazy us) to go out to villages, to the *agraharas* (habitats) of scholars, to look for unpublished manuscripts of great but unhonored or unsung yogis. These would contain enormous information about different yoga practices and experiences of yogis and scholars.

202

❧ DIAGNOSIS ❧

DAVID: In chapter 4 of the *Yoga Rahasya*, the causes and cures of weakness in the body and mind are discussed. Especially in YR IV, 16–19, the text says the causes of weakness may be yoga sadhana, food, not following yama niyama, different parts of the body, nadis and kosas. And, inquiry into these is suggested to discover the exact cause. But, this is no easy matter. How do we go about such an inquiry? Is this a question of having long years of experience so we can find our way? Or, are there some general principles that can guide us?

RAMASWAMI: If yoga is to be used for therapy, the chikitsa karma, the approach of yoga for therapy, will have to be followed. It requires of the therapist that he/she understand the human body—its physiology, the causes of ailments, and the yogic methods for treating them. Several old yoga texts discuss the human body, including the organs (kosas), the energy and other pathways (nadis), and the nodal points (chakras).

In the olden days, the yogis (such as my guru) used to study these topics and work on patients and gain the necessary expertise. But nowadays, even as the practice of asana is popular, study of the ancient texts that describe the nadis, kosas, and chakras is almost nil, as the modern-day yogis and yoga teachers have not learned them. Instead, this lack of knowledge about the body and mind from the yogic perspective is replaced by an extensive study of the human body and mind per the Western system. While this is certainly helpful in making yoga therapy more meaningful, understandable, and applicable in modern times, it also leaves out several methods available in yoga, because they are not intelligible to the modern yoga therapist with his/her Western anatomical knowledge. Most of the research that is going on about the efficacy of the yoga methods is on these modern lines. Although these approaches are welcome, efforts should also be made by serious yoga practitioners to study the ancient system of yoga therapy.

203

SAMANA, UDANA, AND VYANA

DAVID: Are the samana, udana, and vyana vayus (three of the "life forces") of practical use in chikitsa krama?

RAMASWAMI: Samana is the vital force whose *sthana* (position) is in the navel region. It is credited with regularizing the function of digestion. *Sama* = homogenize, *ana* = vital force. So such exercises as kapalabhati and uddiyana bandha, in symmetrical and asymmetrical poses, will help to activate/control this force.

Uda = upward and *ana* = vital force. Udana, situated in the thorax region, is said to control the upward movement of vital ingredients to nourish the brain, and the senses in the head and face. It also controls functions like swallowing. Uddiyana bandha, jalandhara bandha, and the viparita karanis are some of the activities that help energize this force.

Vya = spreading, dispersing; *ana* = vital force. Vyana is the force operating all over the body. It helps circulation of essential fluids for nutrition, prana, and other necessary requirements.

So these are vital forces that would be and should be activated by appropriate yoga practices.

❧ ANATOMY ☙

DAVID: How many anatomical minutiae is it necessary to know for the practice and teaching of yoga? Sometimes, in America, a great deal of anatomy is taught or referred to. Did Krishnamacharya teach this way? I imagine his understanding of anatomy was from the Ayurvedic point of view.

RAMASWAMI: I think a good working knowledge of the anatomical parts and functioning of the body is sufficient to be a successful yoga teacher. My teacher had developed his skills not only by study of the ancient texts but also by his study and observation of his own body and functioning. He had sufficient knowledge to be able to explain everything, even to Western students, with his limited vocabulary of the English language.

During the last twenty years or so, modern yoga, or what you might call Western or American yoga, has taken on a distinctive character. Yoga, with its unique approach to physical culture, had to compete with other popular forms of physical exercise, like gym workouts or even gymnastics. So we have "power yoga" and other similar systems, in which considerable exertion is used, like the pumping and jumping in Ashtanga yoga vinyasas à la gymnastic floor exercises.

Though these were part of the ancient vinyasa yoga, several parameters, such as breathing requirements, keeping the heart rate and breath rate under check, have been passed over in favor of generating excitement. People who want dynamic exercises have found the old yoga a bit too sedate. So, these energetic exercises have drawn a number of enthusiasts to yoga.

Furthermore, many Westerners like to "sweat it out." So, systems of yoga where one is made to profusely sweat by artificially altering the ambient temperature have also become popular.

Another important factor is the therapeutic application of yoga. Along with Ayurveda (the ancient Indian medical system) and other alternative medical systems, yoga has been finding favor as an adjunct therapy. But to validate some of the benefits and also to be acceptable to the Western medical system, Western yoga practitioners have slowly realized the advantage of talking the language of the allopathic medical profession. It is difficult to convince the modern medical system with explanations like "energizing the chakras" or "improving the *prana sanchara* (flow of prana)." With the necessity of getting insurance money for yoga therapy, the system had to bendover backward to make it as intelligible to the Western health people and patients as possible. If you say that the yoga teacher has studied modern anatomy and physiology, it is easier to accept his treatment.

There has also been some research into yoga as a therapy. Several research papers are being published, following the Western research system. And since much of the research is funded by medical institutions, it has become necessary to explain yoga in modern medical terms. Furthermore, the patients and students are more comfortable if the teacher talks about glands and organs rather than kosas and nadis.

I think the Western yoga has come to stay and only a small fraction of the people are really interested in studying yoga in its original version. I feel yoga is slowly becoming a part of Western system, and it is now becoming more and more necessary for the yoga teachers to talk the language of the Western medical man.

In the process many of the lofty and subtle principles of the older yoga system are being lost.

❧ SARVANGASANA ❧

DAVID: Why is sarvangasana so important in chikitsa krama?

RAMASWAMI: Sarvangasana and sirsasana are considered, figuratively and actually, the heart and head of asana practice. As its literal name indicates—all-body-parts pose—sarvangasana is beneficial to all parts of the body, including internal organs. As I have mentioned, according to my teacher, diseases are caused by some of the kosas getting displaced downward from their positions, and daily practice of sarvangasana will help to move the organs in the opposite direction and get them back to their original place. Sarvangasana also helps to relax the muscles of the lower extremities. It helps to reduce pelvic congestion. It helps the heart to rest snugly in the chest cavity (during sarvangasana). Because of natural ujjayi breathing, it will help open the bronchial tubes and dilate them, which will be helpful for those who suffer from bronchial asthma. It can be done even during pregnancy, up to the sixth month or so, as it helps relieve pelvic congestion and reduce edema of the legs. It helps to effectively practice the uddiyana and mula bandhas (due to gravity) and exercise the pelvic organs. For more, please refer to my book *Yoga for the Three Stages of Life*, the section on sarvangasana.

❧ ALLERGIES ❧

DAVID: In the West, many people suffer from allergies. From the point of view of yoga, are allergies viewed as caused by the nadis being clogged or congested so that the prana is not able to flow freely?

RAMASWAMI: To some extent, it may be correct to say that allergies clog the nadis and restrict the healthy functioning of the system. It is especially true of bronchial asthma, in which the passages get constricted and the secretions further clog the pathways.

My guru used to express this graphically. He would say pranayama is like blowing the dirt away from the nadis. So I feel that allergic reactions may become less pronounced if the nadis are cleansed with pranayama. Furthermore, the various exercises of pranayama strengthen the immune system. When you do ujjayi breathing, there is deliberate constriction of the air passages and the sympathetic nervous system gets activated, as it works to open the passages. I have heard a medical doctor say that sarvangasana, due to the nature of the posture, helps one to do ujjayi breathing and strengthens the sympathetic nervous system. This not only helps to open the bronchial tubes, but is also helpful in controlling some related ailments, such as skin allergies like eczema. A lot of research can be done correlating yoga practice, especially pranayama, to the control of allergies.

SLEEP

DAVID: In the commentary to HYP II, 48, Brahmananda quotes a work on yoga describing the daily life of a yogi. Toward the end it states that the yogi should not practice viparita karani in the evening. Is this correct? Somehow I had the impression that sarvangasana was useful in dealing with insomnia and, in that case, you might do it in the evening.

RAMASWAMI: Yes. That is what Brahmananda says. I consider viparita karanai a general term for all inversions. So it could mean a general ban on inversions after sunset. But, in general, my guru did not suggest yoga practice after sunset. In India, evening practice is only done as an exception (I know it is so different in the West). It is customary there to do one's practice in the morning. In case of insomnia, a relaxed viparita karani (a half-shoulder stand) used to be recommended by my guru, as a therapeutic aid. Yes, Brahmananda's view appears to be different.

DAVID: A friend writes: I'm teaching a class, "Yoga for a Good Night's Sleep." Would you kindly suggest some practices?

RAMASWAMI: Good stretching vinyasas, especially of the arms and upper body with slow, smooth, long breaths in standing or lying-down position; sarvangasana or viparita karani, with the legs kept nicely relaxed for a few minutes with normal breathing; a few kapalabhatis followed by short inhalations and very long smooth exhalations; shanmukhi mudra, with the mind following the breath; chanting or listening to the peace chants or some good music should be helpful.

DAVID: Can yoga offer any help with the problem of sleep apnea?

RAMASWAMI: First, we need to check the breath. Getting the breath free and smooth, with long inhale and exhale, might help.

Beyond this, yoga has very limited methods that may be tried. One is simhasana-type breathing, where you open the mouth (throat) wide and stretch the tongue out and breathe. (This breathing is explained in *Yoga for the Three Stages of Life*.) This may be practiced regularly to strengthen the lax throat tissues. About six breaths, two to three times a day, especially before going to bed, may be attempted.

Another procedure would be to do ujjayi breathing in sarvangasana, or an easier version of viparita karani. The idea is to practice ujjayi breathing with a good jalandhara bandha, which becomes possible in viparita karani.

A few rounds of kapalabhati may also be helpful. (Sinus problems have to be cured first, before kapalabhati.)

Loud chanting of Omkara may also be attempted.

❧ KAPALABHATI ❧

DAVID: A question from a friend: Is the kapalabhati kriya (rapid abdominal breathing) good for a beginning cold with some chest congestion?

RAMASWAMI: Kapalabhati usually clears the whole breathing passage and, if done regularly, will help one to breathe freely and easily, preventing colds and or other respiratory problems. In the case of those who are new to kapalabhati, one has to see if the nose is congested, in which case it may be better to avoid kapalabhati, as sometimes people tend to force the secretions into the sinuses.

If it is just the beginning of a cold and if the student has done kapalabhati before, you may suggest Kapalabhati a few times, say about twenty-four times, repeated two or three times a day. Another option would be to do sarvangasana or, better, viparita karani, and stay for a few minutes. There is an increased blood supply to the face (especially in viparita karani) and it may help to relieve the congestion to some extent.

DAVID: A colleague writes: "I find the effects of kapalabhati calming and lightening. Last week, I taught it to eight cancer patients (following their asana practice) at a hospital. I only had them do about six to eight breaths, to watch for tension in neck and jaw area, not to be too forceful nor too rapid—in other words not to overexert the nervous system. I asked them to describe what they experienced. They felt more heated and clearer—they liked it. Cancer patients are usually cold."

Would kapalabhati be approved of by Krishnamacharya and yourself in these circumstances—or should I not be teaching this to cancer patients?

RAMASWAMI: I think patients recovering from cancer can use kapalabhati. It is an enlivening procedure. The test should be whether the person is able to feel well and comfortable after the brief stint of kapalabhati. It could be too much for a few who are really sick, and the guidance should be quite involved.

DAVID: A colleague writes: "The medical encyclopedia defines *hyperventilation* in the following way: 'Hyperventilation is rapid or deep breathing, usually caused by anxiety or panic. This overbreathing, as it is sometimes called, actually leaves you feeling breathless.'

"When you breathe, you inhale oxygen and exhale carbon dioxide. Excessive breathing leads to low levels of carbon dioxide in your blood, which causes many of the symptoms that you may feel if you hyperventilate.

"Since breath is forced out of the lungs by the exaggerated upper movement of the diaphragm in kapalabhati and bhastrika, it seems that a more than usual amount of carbon dioxide would be expelled. How, then, is kapalabhati or bastrika different from hyperventilation?"

RAMASWAMI: The literal meaning of the term *hyperventilation* is "excess breathing," and one can apply that term to kapalabhati. In kapalabhati, the rate of breathing is four to five times the rate of normal breathing, and there is certainly increased ventilation.

But then, medically, the term hyperventilation is used in a condition with an underlying pathology or psychological factor. In such cases, hyperventilation occurs to correct some pathology, such as acidosis. But while practicing kapalabhati, even though there is a reduction in the carbon dioxide level in the blood, it is usually within normal limits (except when you overdo it). In fact many, at the end of practicing kapalabhati for a minute or two, experience a suspension of breath, associated with a very pleasant feeling for a very short duration, before normal breathing starts; whereas, in the case of medical condition of hyperventilation, there is uncontrolled, anxious breathing. Such breathing looks not at all like kapalabhati.

A few years ago, I was doing a one-semester yoga program for the medical students in Ramachandra Medical University, in India. A student compared kapalabhati to hyperventilation. The professor of physiology, who was also attending the program, immediately pointed out that the way kapalabhati is done is so different from the breathing that takes place in a patient who may be hyperventilating, and added that kapalabhati cannot be compared to hyperventilation.

Kapalabhati, like neti and other kriyas, is a cleansing process. In medical hyperventilation, there exists a precondition that requires correction. In kapalabhati, by controlled, rapid, deep breathing for a short period of time, the system rids itself of excess toxins (such as carbon dioxide), bringing the system into a healthy range.

❧ TERMINAL ILLNESS ❧

DAVID: A friend writes: "The yoga philosophy I have studied so far (and I am only a beginner) talks about living correctly and keeping the body healthy as a precondition or as part of the practices that ultimately quiet the mind. What does yoga say about someone who has a sick body (a condition that cannot be cured or alleviated)? From the yoga viewpoint, can they ever find tranquility?"

RAMASWAMI: Yoga philosophy talks not only about asanas, but also about other aspects. In fact, if a person is sick or old or cannot do asanas, Kriya yoga (yoga of action) can be attempted. It basically requires the patient to have control over the senses, like eating, speaking, and so on. Study of an appropriate philosophy, devotional poems or hymns, chanting, or anything that uplifts the spirit can be tried. Then, if the patient is religiously inclined, a positive direction can be given to this attitude by study of the appropriate scriptures; specific devotional practices can be attempted. With Kriya yoga, Patanjali says, one can greatly reduce the mental pain (klesha tanukarana) of illness.

212

❧ UNEVEN HIPS ❧

DAVID: What is chikitsa krama for someone with uneven hips? I imagine sarvangasana would be helpful. But do adaptations need to be made in seated or squatting poses, such as ardha-uttanasana, uttanasana, or paschimatanasana?

RAMASWAMI: If the body is uneven, we have to use different adaptive movements for either side separately, and so asymmetrical seated vinyasas will be helpful. The purpose should be to exercise the different parts of the body, including the affected part. These exercises may not be helpful in correcting the malformation. The use of a judicious combination of vinyasas will be helpful to some extent in growing children, when their age may make it possible to achieve some correction of the deformities of the spine, hip, or other bones. The asanas you have mentioned will be helpful to exercise those joints that may not be properly exercised in the normal course of events.

DAVID: Is there some risk to them in doing symmetrical asanas? Should one exclude uttanasana, paschimatanasana, or similar poses completely and stick to just the asymmetrical ones as you recommend? What of the forward bending and squatting in the tadasana sequence—are these not appropriate?

RAMASWAMI: As a rule, if there is unevenness, symmetrical poses will produce uneven stretch. So we have to see each condition and come up with a regimen that will be suitable. In asymmetrics, you can isolate one joint or group of muscles and work on the other. I think it will also depend upon the degree of unevenness. If it is imperceptible—as most of us have some asymmetry—then the even stretches can be used. But if it is significant, then uttanasana and paschimatanasana may be avoided.

I remember my guru mentioning that asymmetrics like triang mukha (backward facing) could be useful for persons with partially amputated lower extremities.

213

❦ TRACHEOTOMY ❦

DAVID: Yesterday, I was approached about seeing a student who has had a tracheotomy. This is the operation that involves slitting open the windpipe and inserting a tube so the person can breathe when his upper respiratory tract is blocked.

Of course, I want to help. But I feel I'm over my head here. Use of the breath is such a big element of our yoga. Here there may still be some breathing through the nose and mouth, but mostly he's breathing through this artificial opening.

Do you have any experience or recommendations for how to proceed in this case? I would certainly appreciate any advice.

RAMASWAMI: I think without a firsthand observation of the patient, it may not be possible to suggest anything. If the patient has some voluntary control over his breathing, maybe some arm movements with a little longer breathing may help, but is the patient in that condition? Another difficulty could be the tube inserted for breathing. Perhaps with some movements it may get disturbed, creating problems, especially if he has other tubes or devices inserted as well. Maybe with more detailed information we can think of something that could be useful.

❧ DENTAL PROBLEMS ❧

DAVID: Next week I'm having (minor) oral surgery—a tooth extraction. They've recommended no physical activity for a week. I think this is a bit of an exaggeration, as I will be allowed to walk and drive my car. Still, I'm thinking of modifying my yoga practice as follows: As far as the asanas are concerned: no inversions, no forward bends where the head goes below the waist, and no desk pose. As for my pranayama practice, no pushing the inhale and no hold after inhale. So, I'm thinking of practicing a few arm movements and exhale pranayama. Any advice you could offer would be greatly appreciated.

RAMASWAMI: Some people experience considerable pain and some have some bleeding problem after dental surgery, so it is safer not to strain by doing exercises that may aggravate the problems.

6

On Everyday Matters

INTRODUCTION

WHAT IS THE role of yoga in everyday life?

The ultimate goal of yoga is freedom (kaivalya), but it is a long-term one. Still, if we head toward this goal, along the way we acquire health, stability, and clarity of mind. These are invaluable in everyday life. So why not use yoga to achieve these positive qualities?

Most people today take up yoga not for the ultimate goal of freedom, but to reduce their stress, stay in good health, and gain clarity of mind so that they can pursue the goals of their everyday life, not the goal of yoga. Many people take up yoga for exercise only and it meets this purpose. Some people try and read the *Yoga Sutras* as a guide to how to live their everyday life. But this is not the purpose for which it was written. Still, it has so much to teach us about our minds that many find it useful in everyday life. So maybe yoga *can* be viewed as a guide for everyday living.

Yoga, Samkhya, and Vedanta all have a spiritual goal. If we lose sight of it, much of what these schools say becomes irrelevant. There is a saying I am fond of, "If a man does not know to which port he is sailing, no wind is favorable to him." Yoga basically would say that the spirit/self/indwelling nonchanging consciousness is the principle that qualifies to be called "I," and not the ever-changing mind-body complex as we normal mortals believe. If the mind can transform itself by yoga practice to remain firmly in this state, and shift the focus from the physical to the spiritual self, it achieves freedom because the person knows—not just believes—that he/she is immortal.

But many with the immediate concerns of day-to-day life cannot find solace in this goal, not at the moment. But if they still want help from yoga to reduce the pain of attachments, aversions, or fear, has yoga anything to offer? With the ultimate goal in the back of one's mind, if one takes to yoga, life becomes lot more purposeful, and living it very practical.

In Patanjali's *Yoga Sutras*, in the commentary of Vyasa, at the end of the discourse on yoga and kaivalya in the first chapter, the student demurs and asks, "It is okay for people with a balanced mind to pursue yoga with the highest goal in mind, but what of us, the millions whose minds are constantly looking outward to the external world for happiness and satisfaction?" Patanjali offers Kriya yoga for such earnest people who want to reduce the pain that most of us seem to experience most of the time. Kriya yoga basically is yoga of action or activities to clean up the body and mind.

What are the components of Kriya yoga, which one can put into practice on a day-to-day basis?

First, it is moderation, or *tapas*. It is to keep everything that we take in under check—what we eat, what we hear and see and experience from the outside world. The senses should not be clogged. My guru would say that food, entertainment, communication, and interaction with others and the outside world should be under moderation. This gives considerable free space to the mind, and one will start feeling less stressed. As is commonly said, one should be able to say no after a while, be it to entertainment, food, small talk, or involvement in outside activity. It gives more time for contemplation, reflection, and refinement. Walking, practice of asanas and many vinyasas, and breathing exercises will also be necessary. My teacher used to advise my parents when there were not practicing yoga regularly, "Please do some vyayama [regular exercises]."

Second, one should spend time on studies—study of authentic yoga books that give more theoretical information about yoga. If I wanted to be a physicist or a physician, I would have to study the appropriate books to get the necessary knowledge to be able to successfully practice. So if I want to use/practice yoga to uplift myself, I must spend some time studying yoga on a regular basis. Practice and study should go hand in hand. One without the other is futile. So, all those who have taken to yoga must start studying yoga. Chanting has a very soothing effect on the mind. I always liked chanting. I still fondly remember the hundreds of hours of chanting I have done with my guru. My mother once said, after an hour's chanting in my house, that just listening to chanting of the Vedas had a salutary effect on the mind and moods. Svadhyaya (study) and chanting can be an important mind-cleansing process.

People are caught up with the tensions of the complicated day-to-day modern life. In this world, people who have innate faith in God are really blessed. Prayer and worship of God, Isvarapranidhana, in whatever method one is used to, can make the difference between stress and sanity. Isvarapranidhana is a positive practice that yoga recommends to those who have the faith.

There are other yamas and niyamas that one could try to follow faithfully. Constant remembrance of these and diligent practices slowly transforms the mind and replaces old unhealthy and stressful samskaras (habits) with wholesome, positive, and peaceful ones.

217

Patanjali would say that if one follows these simple practices, one will develop a positive state of mind. By following Kriya yoga, the mental pain that one experiences will reduce substantially. It does not take place in one day, but the benefits do manifest in a short time of steady practice.

✌ CONSCIENCE ✌

DAVID: Conscience. The little voice within. The voice that tells us right from wrong. I don't know if you have this concept in India. In Western religions, it is often regarded as the personal interface between man and God—the divine voice inside us telling us what is morally correct according to God's law. But what can this be in Patanjali's system? Conscience is just another samskara. It may be a mental habit from childhood; it may arise from a *vasana* (latent residual memory) from a past life. But, it cannot be the "voice" of purusha. It cannot be the "voice" of Isvara. Or can it?

RAMASWAMI: In Samkhya and yoga, it will be the samskara of dharma, which the yogi has developed here or here before, which will be the guiding light. However, Isvarapranidhana can develop this. Since the Lord, Isvara, has all the knowledge and is also the primary preceptor, surrendering to him will enable the yogi to acquire the dharmic samskaras to enable him to lead the uplifting dharmic life.

But, generally speaking, the Vedic religion also recognizes God as the Inner self (*antaratma* or *antaryami*, the inner guide or controller). In my language, the term used for God is *Kadavul*, which literally means the principle that is deepest inside us.

❧ GOD IS EVERYWHERE ❧

DAVID: If we follow a religious belief that God is present everywhere in creation, then we would believe that life is divine, that the body is divine, and our very breath is a gift from the Divine. If we believe that life and the body are divine, why not live life fully and enjoy the pleasures of the body and the intimate connections with others? Why not find joy in the divine life granted us? After all, the pain and suffering are due to avidya, misconception. Why view the body and its relationships as obstacles to be transcended? True, the body decays as we age, but, if we accept the body as a manifestation of the Divine, why consider it disgusting (Vyasa's commentary on YS II, 5)?

RAMASWAMI: Even as God created everything and is omnipresent, he also has given out, in the scriptures, the rules (dharma) by which to live correctly, called. If I do things that are not dharma, it is also ordained by God that I will suffer the consequences. So the rules and commandments of the Divine will have to be followed. God wants the devotee to uplift from the state of tamas to rajas to satwa and then beyond the three gunas, as Lord Krishna instructs Arjuna (*nis traigunya bhava Arjuna*) in the Bhagavad Gita. God, as the *Yoga Sutras* say, also gives you the correct knowledge about the nature of the body and the nature of the self. So, per the texts, the body is not the self, and the persistence to consider the body as the self, which is avidya, will have to be overcome. That is the knowledge Isvara, or God, gives when you pray to him for knowledge, spiritual knowledge.

There is an interesting statement made by Lord Krishna. He says, inter alia, that everything is in him but he is not in everything. This implies that, though God created the universe and permeates it, if you are looking to know God, then he can be found only in certain places—say, in the purity (satwa) of the devotee's heart. God is everywhere, but divinity does not manifest everywhere.

✿ RELIGION AND YOGA Q&A ✿

DAVID: I am not a Hindu, but a follower of the Jewish tradition. Is there any conflict between my religious practices and yoga?

RAMASWAMI: As the *Yoga Sutras* say, and according to my teacher, a yogi should follow his/her own religious practices (*yeta abhimata dhyanat va*). So swadhyaya, as it is explained from my religious background in my book *Yoga for the Three Stages of Life*, should be understood to mean authentic religious and philosophical studies. I am sure there can be no conflict between studying and practicing yoga and being deeply faithful to one's own religion.

✿ DESPAIR ✿

DAVID: When I study the *Yoga Sutras* and read your answers to my questions, I realize that many of the things we talk about are out of reach in this lifetime. Even the most basic things, such as stopping the mind from wandering, seem extraordinarily difficult. So, my question is, how far can I go? And, if it is so unlikely that I will reach kaivalya, should I even bother with the practice? What is to be gained? Is it the reduction of pain? Is that really the practical idea?

RAMASWAMI: This is exactly the trap of despair into which one should not fall. If one develops these feelings of despair even with mundane things, one is likely to be pulled down. So what can we say about spiritual matters?

The basic question to be answered is, "Have I started the inward journey and am I progressing on the right lines?" A journey of a thousand miles starts with but a single step. *Yoga Sutras* talk about it, in YS I, 20–22. One should be earnest, whole-heartedly engaged in yogic practice, and direct one's entire energy into it. Some put mild effort, some moderate, and some full application. Kaivalya may take place in this birth or in some future birth.

There is a book called *Kaivalya Navaneetha* in my mother   221 tongue. It is said to be a wonderful book on Vedanta. The title means "Butter of Freedom." Butter was a favorite edible item with children in the olden days. It means the book talks about kaivalya being as happiness-giving as is butter to a child. Another understanding of this metaphor is that, if the yogi is sufficiently evolved to obtain the spiritual freedom, the time taken can be as small as the time taken to swallow a piece of butter. Or it could mean that by reading the book there will be so much clarity that the reader will get kaivalya as easily as swallowing butter.

Here is a small story. Once there was a yogi who spent all his time in the practice of yoga, but was concerned about the time that he would take to attain kaivalya. One day as he was doing yoga practice, a renowned sage passed that way. The yogi asked the sage to observe his practice and tell him the time that it would take for him to get the ultimate result. The sage showed the yogi a nearby tree with plenty of branches and leaves, and said that it may take as many lives as there were leaves in the tree. The *yogabhyasi* (practitioner) was naturally upset, but pointed to another person who was just sitting under the tree but who appeared uncon-cerned about anything. He asked the sage, how long will it take for the other person to achieve kaivalya? The sage pointed to another tree in which there was just one leaf. As the sage smiled, a mild wind blew and the only leaf fell off, to indicate that the other one was a successful yogi.

No despair, no concerns in spiritual practice. These are the exact chitta vrittis (mental projections) we would like to overcome.

❦ COMPARISONS ❧

DAVID: Comparisons are odious, yet we make them all the time. Is the next person richer than I am? Smarter than I am? Stronger than I am? Can he do more asanas than me? Is his breath longer than mine? We even do this in the spiritual realm: Is this person closer to God than I am? Has he reached a higher level than I have? We even make comparisons with ourselves: Was my practice today better, deeper than yesterday? Was my meditation stronger? Comparisons may make us feel good (briefly) or bad. But, aren't they a sign that we are not content? Are there specific practices that can help us acquire santosha (contentment), which is, after all, one of the niyamas?

RAMASWAMI: Patanjali mentions that the klesha vrittis (pain-provoking thoughts) should be reduced by dhyana (complete concentration). A proper understanding of the Karma theory, the nature of the self, the predominance of duhkha (pain) in the cycle of births and deaths, will create the correct attitude of contentment in the mind of the yogabhyasi. A strong theoretical understanding is sufficient and necessary to be able to get to a stage of santosha. In the earlier Kriya yoga, swadhyaya is mentioned prominently. Then santosha becomes possible. A yogic bent of mind is perhaps necessary.

❦ MEMORIES ❧

DAVID: Memory (*smirti*) is such a powerful force in our lives. Memories of childhood, memories of loved ones—these seem to stay with us always, affecting our thoughts and our actions. Are there specific practices to cleanse the memory or weaken the grip these memories have on us? Or is this just something that happens along the way, on the road to kaivalya?

222

RAMASWAMI: Childhood experiences vary from person to person. Some have a reasonably good childhood and have generally pleasant memories. Some others may have been traumatized, and these memories haunt them. But, according to Patanjali, once the subject knows and realizes that the true nature of the self is consciousness and consciousness alone, and all the experiences pertain to the mind and do not affect the self (it is a tall order but, according to Patanjali's *Yoga Sutras*, it is the reality), then he/she is able to look at the past and present more objectively.

223

Kaivalya comes only from the understanding of the self—one's own self. Even before kaivalya takes place, the attitude of the yogi toward the events of the past and his/her reactions to them will undergo a sea change. The transformation will have to take place. After practicing, studying, and contemplating on the principles of yoga, there will be an attitudinal change toward the past memories.

CONFLICT

DAVID: Conflict. It always agitates the mind. How do we deal with it? Arjuna, in the Bhagavad Gita, was instructed to fight. It was his dharma. He was a soldier. We may not be. Should we always walk away from conflict? *Upekshanam* (avoidance) suggests we ignore people who do evil, that we not have any associations with them. We might call them "toxic people" and try our best to avoid them, not have them be part of our lives. But, not all conflicts can be avoided. As long as we are involved with other people, conflicts are inevitable. There are times when a person may be attacking our livelihood or our family. Then we must fight. Or, so it seems. And then there are times when we just feel we must stand up for ourselves to receive our just credit, our due rewards. Perhaps at these times we should be practicing Isvarapranidhana, placing the fruits of our labors at the feet of the Lord.

RAMASWAMI: One important concept we have to consider, in all these, is to determine: whom is this addressed to? This is called *adhikari bheda*, or the difference in the persons who can follow certain procedures. The case of Arjuna and the case of the *uttama adhikara* (the most fit person for yoga), mentioned in the *Yoga Sutras*, where upeksha also is referred to, are different. Arjuna's dharma, as the commander in chief of the army, was to fight at that time. But he chose to run away from his duty. Can a soldier refuse to fight on a battlefield, leave alone the commander in chief, exposing his own buddies to the danger of annihilation? Normally, such a person would be subjected to court-martial. Sometimes I wonder how Arjuna could think of running away from battle at all. If he had wanted no war, he should have taken to *sanyasa* (renunciation, the spiritual way of life), without working with his brothers and allies up to the stage of a final war, which according to the Mahabharata was a just war (*dharma yuddha*). Just as Arjuna had some duties to perform, so do people like us: family men, teachers, and others.

According to conventional wisdom, Arjuna's condition is typical of that of most people. Each has responsibilities, toward the family, nation, work, society, and others. All of one's duties will have to be fulfilled. After one discharges one's responsibilities, one can take fully to spiritual life. In the olden days, one may not have been able to take to sanyasa without the explicit permission of the spouse, as happened in the case of Yagnyavalkya, or one's mother, as in the cases of Patanjali and Adi Sankara.

Doing one's duty without hankering after rewards or recognition typifies the attitude of a Karma yogi, which is to do prescribed duties. Most householders should be Karma yogis if they want to tread the spiritual path. As mentioned, once the duties are discharged, one can take fully to spiritual life, renouncing the life of a householder. Taking to spiritual life prematurely is fraught with danger. On the other hand, many people, even after they have adequately discharged their duties, cling to materialistic life.

The Upeksha-practicing yogi, referred to in Patanjali's *Yoga Sutras*, develops the samskara of avoiding "toxic people" situations. The yogi does not harbor any illusions of his/her being out there to transform the world, but is after his/her own liberation, or kaivalya. For ordinary mortals like us, it may not be completely possible, but we can keep this advice at the back of our mind. We need not subjugate ourselves and our families to the dictates of adharmic people. However, we can make a definite effort to reduce such associations.

225

Once a yogi was passing through a village, where a powerful thug was terrorizing everyone. But when the thug saw the yogi, he felt a tender feeling and begged the yogi to reform him. The yogi advised him to practice ahimsa, the minimum requirement of a yogi. After the passage of considerable time, the yogi again passed that way, only to find even street urchins throwing stones at the once-powerful thug, now a weakling. The yogi saw what had happened. The man had taken the yogi's advice literally, and had meekly submitted himself to all abuses without retaliating. That was his understanding of ahimsa. Everyone, including the weakest, felt emboldened to attack the man. The yogi then said to him that what he told him was not to attack anyone, but did not say that he should not defend himself. He said to him, "You can raise the stick to threaten and drive away your attackers, without actually striking." So upeksha is not such an impractical advice. Even sanyasins, as they go through the forests, carry a long stick to scare away wild animals who cross their path.

❧ DEATH ❧

DAVID: In YY X, 19–20, Yagnavalkya says that whatever we think at the time of death will be what we become. I assume this means we become that in our next birth. It sounds magical. Can we really control our rebirth with just our final thought? And, how does it work? Suppose we hold our mind on our personal deity at the end. Surely, we don't become that.

RAMASWAMI: Yes, if we could control our thoughts and think what we desire at the time of death to influence our next birth, it would be wonderful. But it is also true that, at the time of death, our thoughts are dominated by our samskaras. A person who, all his/her life, been feeling unfulfilled and angry, will not be able to remain peaceful at the time of death. It is customary to say that one should develop dharmic thoughts all through life so that, at the time of death, due to samskaras, those thoughts alone will dominate the mind. I think it's impossible to control the thoughts at the time of death. The dominant samskara will take over, as mentioned in the Karma theory in the *Yoga Sutras*. As in dreams, we lose control of our thoughts. At the time of death, thoughts cannot be controlled.

There is a story about a devotee of the Lord, who, during his prayers, would say, "I may not be able to remember you at the time of death. So consider my thoughts of you that I have right now as my final thoughts."

Usually, the person concerned considers the personal deity as the ultimate reality. So when someone thinks of the Lord at the time of death, he or she is supposed to go to heaven or the abode of the Lord. Here again, there are different kinds of results. If you think of the Lord and have his form in your mind, after death you attain a form similar to him (*sarupya*). If you see yourself remaining in his abode (heaven [*saloka*]), you will reach that abode. If you see yourself standing in front of the Lord and look at his divine form, you will be in his world, having the vision of the Lord all the time, looking at him (*samipya*). On the other hand, if you imagine yourself as completely losing yourself in him, like a drop of water falling into the ocean, you become merged in him (*sayujya*), which, according to Bhakti yogis is *moksha* (the ultimate release).

DAVID: I have a friend who is going through a difficult emotional period. A member of her family has been diagnosed with cancer. It is very upsetting. And, naturally, my friend's mind is quite distracted. Is it right to suggest she keep up her yoga practice? I think it could be a great help to her. On the other hand, since her mind is distracted, she is not able to focus on the breath. Still, some practice of asana, even very strong asana, may help to reduce the disturbance, quiet the mind some, and then she will be able to continue with a more focused mind.

227

RAMASWAMI: In my immediate family, three members in the recent past were struck by cancer. The spouses of the patients reacted in a similar way. They were shocked and stunned at the suddenness and the gravity of the situation. But they quickly regrouped themselves, accepted the help of friends and relatives, consulted the doctors, and did their best to be supportive of the ailing spouses. For the next several months, they maintained their composure, giving all their attention, care, and love they could to the spouse. When negative thoughts about the worst scenario plagued their minds, they prayed, harnessed their mental resources, and did what best they could do physically, financially, emotionally for the patient. Sooner than later, they said to themselves that what they should do was to do their best and leave the rest to God (or fate). One of the close relatives was cured completely, but the other two did not survive. There was grief, but the enduring feeling that medically, emotionally, and financially, the best had been done, and a feeling of surrender to the grand scheme of things helped them to get over the grief in a short period of time.

In such situations, a tamasic mind goes into depression; the rajasic frets, fumes, or overreacts; but the satwic composes itself and does what is best for the situation (dharma) and remains focused. When one is an outsider to the immediate situation, we have to find what practice would be helpful to the person close to the patient. It could be prayer, mantra chant, asana practice, reading, taking help from a good support group, or anything that will give confidence or ekagrata (one-pointedness). I would first talk to the friend and find out what aspect of yoga would be helpful. As you say, it could be asana practice, or reading, or listening to music that is comforting to the person concerned. Several methods of ekagrata are mentioned in YS I, 33, such as long and complete exhalation, retention of breath after exhalation, imaging a spot of light in the heart, religious practice, and visiting saintly persons.

228

❧ RAMANUJA ❧

DAVID: I was reading a short biography of Ramanuja (a scholar) and came across the story of how his first teacher, Yadava, feared that Ramanuja would become a dualist and, in time, an opponent of advaita. So, Yadava decided it was best to do away with Ramanuja. After Ramanuja was murdered, Yadava thought he could wash off the sin by a bath in the holy Ganges. I could hardly believe it. Is the philosophy one holds so important that one could take another's life over it? How could an esteemed teacher of Vedanta even consider murder? It is true that the plot was foiled and that later Yadava recanted and became Ramanuja's student, but still, that he even conceived the plot was upsetting. But then I thought about how many religious wars there have been in the West. How many killings there have been in the name of God. And, then I thought, well, this is just more of the same. Hard to believe, but it goes on all the time.

RAMASWAMI: Yes, when one's beliefs are threatened, one becomes shaky and loses composure. Sometimes the response is violent. When two people debate a point, the first sign of losing an argument is the show of seething anger. My guru once quoted a famous saying, "*Sesham kopena purayeth*"—"The rest was made up of anger."

A frail scholar went for a debate. He argued so well that the opponent could not find a suitable counterargument. He beat the frail scholar to submission. The thug-debater won the debate by filling the remainder of the debate with anger.

229

Ramanuja was about to be harmed. Some sects of Tantric religious practice have physically harmed Adi Sankara. I think more people have been killed in the name of faith than for any other cause. These days, we see a lot of angry action in almost all fields: politics, business, and, perhaps to a very small extent, even yoga.

But some of the stories, I feel, are exaggerated. These storywriters tend to exaggerate some events favoring their hero and putting the adversary in a poor light. It is sad that religion and philosophy, which should give happiness and peace, sometimes create the opposite effect.

❧ NETI POT ❧

DAVID: Do you recommend the use of the neti pot (a cleansing process)?

RAMASWAMI: In his book *Yoga Makaranda*, My teacher included the use of neti kriya for cleansing purposes. But he never taught this to me. Among the kriyas (yogic cleansing procedures), he encouraged us to do only kapalabhati kriya (rapid abdominal breathing). He indicated that this was necessary and sufficient, and felt introducing other foreign elements into the body through nose is not necessary. *Hatha Yoga Pradipika* also suggests that these kriyas are optional practices, which can be used in case of impurities (*malas*) in the body.

∞ WALKING ∞

DAVID: Do you recommend walking to students? I find walking quite helpful in dealing with digestion and the emotions. I've started to wonder if it shouldn't be considered part of a yoga practice. I think in India, especially in times past, before there were cars, people must have walked a great deal. Krishnamacharya seems to have walked all over the country. So, I wonder if it was just assumed that students would be walking a lot. I never see it mentioned in the texts.

RAMASWAMI: As you say, Indians of yesteryear traveled a lot by foot. My guru used to suggest walking. As mentioned earlier, he would also say that one should walk with a straight back, but the head slightly down, looking at the ground ahead of one. One must plant the feet fully on the ground while one walks. When he walked, his feet also were straight and not opened out as many people walk. He had talked about walking around the streets of Mysore, chanting Vedic hymns for the infirm in the houses to hear. Mahatma Gandhi was a brisk and relentless walker. The much revered Kanchi Sankaracharya (head of the monastery in Kanchi), who lived for a hundred years, walked all over the country in the twentieth century.

Sanyasins are not supposed to stay in one place for more than three nights (*tri ratram*). So the sanyasins are committed walkers. In the olden days, one of the vows of many orthodox people was to visit several holy shrines, and places like Varanashi in the north and Rameshwar in the South, necessitating years of travel by walking. The old and the infirm may have been carried in carts or palanquins, but the majority of the ancient people walked.

While my teacher would walk and suggest walking, he was against other forms of physical exercise, such as jogging or other sports activities. He would say these strain the system unequally and could be harmful. A yogabhyasi has to be careful not to injure himself. He should not take part in sports and other recreational activities that have an element of danger.

✳ TRAVEL ✳

DAVID: How do you adjust your practice when traveling? When there is less time and perhaps more agitation?

RAMASWAMI: It is certainly difficult. Since we do not walk to our destination, it may be a good idea to stop the vehicle after a few hours of driving and walk for about ten minutes. One may do some stretching vinyasas in tadasana. One asana that will help to relieve congestion in your legs, due to sitting while driving or traveling by plane, is sarvangasana. One may be a spectacle in an airport, but maybe will start a new trend. Five to ten minutes in sarvangasana or viparita karani, and a few leg movements in it, will be very helpful. While waiting for the connecting flight in the hub airport, I try to walk in the airport. Sitting up and doing shanmukhi mudra for about five minutes, observing the breath, would lead to considerable reduction in anxiety.

✳ HAPPINESS ✳

DAVID: Was Krishnamacharya happy at the end of his life?

RAMASWAMI: Was he happy? Maybe he was. Was he contented (*santosha*)? Yes, he was, I would guess. If a man could worship the Lord with the same fervor at the age of ninety-nine as he was doing at the age of sixty-six, he must have been a contented man. If a man can teach with the same conviction and sincerity at the age of ninety-nine as he was teaching at the age of sixty-six, he should be at peace with himself. At ninety-nine, if a man could chant the scriptures from memory, lying down in his bed (he was incapacitated due to a fall), as he used to do when he was hale and healthy at sixty-six, he must have been a happy man.

He had many ups and downs in his life. To relocate at the age of sixty-six, to support a large family, starting life all over again in a new place, would upset anybody. His absolute faith in the Lord, and the conviction that one should do one's duty (*swadharma*), was uppermost in his mind. His understanding of the scriptures, and the conviction that they are the messages of the Lord, guided his whole life. I thought he considered that teaching the scriptures and living by their dictates were the main concerns of life. Every generation throws out teachers who would faithfully impart the knowledge and dharma to the next generation. I think he felt that his duty was to impart that knowledge; and by such activities he was fulfilling his life's goal, consistent with the dictates of the Lord.

I am sure he was at peace with himself, supported perhaps emotionally by his devotion to the Lord, intellectually by his understanding of the scriptures and his sincere commitment to teaching, even as he would appear stern and sometimes uncompromising.

Studying with Sri. T. Krishnamacharya

SRIVATSA RAMASWAMI'S GURU, Sri. T. Krishnamacharya, taught not only yoga and the various aspects of yoga, but also several other related orthodox philosophies. He was a qualified teacher of nyaya, the powerful system of logic used for spiritual discussions in olden times. He was known as Nyayacharya. He taught *Nyaya Sutras* and *Tarka Samgraha*, two important ancient works related to this subject. He taught Vedic chanting extensively, and was given a title Veda Kesaari (Lion of the Vedas). He not only chanted with a booming voice but also taught the Vedic philosophy related to the ritualistic portion, known as Mimamsa. He taught Samkhya as well, and obtained a diploma in this philosophy, for these achievements he was known by the title Samkhya Siromani (crest jewel of Samkhya). Of course he was also known as Yogacharya. He taught the Upanishads, the Bhagavad Gita and the Brahma Sutras, the important three sets of texts for the Vedic philosophy known as Vedanta, and earned the title Vedanta Vageesa, meaning the "master exponent of Vedanta." He could teach with equal facility the Advaitic and Visishtadvaitic interpretation of Vedanta, even as he favored Ramanuja's Visishtadwaitic interpretation. Apart from these Vedic subjects and philosophies, he also was a scholar of the great epic *Ramayana* (story of Rama) and other mythologies such as *Vishnu Purana, Bhagavata Purana* (Story of Lord Krishna), as well as several other Vaishnavite religious texts. He taught these subjects individually depending upon the requirements of each student. Because of his vast studies and knowledge, he had a very comprehensive view of the whole range of Eastern philosophies and religious practices, and guided his students according to what he thought was the appropriate path for each. Yogis who would like to enlarge their knowledge base of spirituality, may wish to study more of these texts, slowly, one by one.

Bibliography

Yoga Sutras of Patanjali (YS)
There are countless translations and commentaries of this ancient text. Two
we recommend are:

Yoga Philosophy of Patanjali, with the commentary of Hariharananda
Aranya (University of Calcutta, 2000). This book very closely follows tradition. The translation and copious notes add value to the book.

Patanjali's Yoga Sutras: Based on the Teaching of Srivatsa Ramaswami by
Pamela Hoxsey (tel.: 1-847-328-4246). This book contains word by word
meaning and paraphrase of all the Sutras and some notes. It also contains
an audio CD with the beautiful chanting of the entire *Yoga Sutras*, by Pam
Hoxsey.

Yoga Rahasya (Secret of Yoga) of Nathamuni (YR)
T. Krishnamacharya; T. K. V. Desikachar, trans. Krishnamacharya Yoga
Mandiram, Revised Edition, 2003. Was inspired by Krishnamacharya's devo-
tion to Nathamuni.

Hatha Yoga Pradipika (HYP)
Svatmarama, with the commentary of Brahmananda. Adyar Library edition,
Adyar Library, 1972

Yoga for the Three Stages of Life (YTSL)
Srivatsa Ramaswami. Inner Traditions, 2000.

Complete Book of Vinyasa Yoga (CBVY)
Srivatsa Ramaswami. Marlowe & Co., 2005.

The Yoga Yajnavalkya (YY)
A. G. Mohan, trans. Ganesh & Co. of Madras.

Yoga Makaranda
T. Krishnamacharya; T. K. V. Desikachar, trans. Serialized in the magazine
KYM Darsanam, 1994–96.

Suggestions
for Further Reading

(See *Yoga for the Three Stages of Life*, chapter 15, Yoga Texts, for guidance and further suggestions)

Samkhya Karika—Core text of philosophy fundamental to understanding yoga. Samkhya, along with yoga and Vedanta, was considered an orthodox philosophy of the Vedas, leading to ultimate release of the soul from bondage. The commentaries by Gaudapada and Vacaspati Misra are considered very authentic, and English translations are available.

Bhagavad Gita—This great text from the epic *Mahabharata* is a treatise on yoga, Vedanta, and dharma. Considered to be one of the foremost works, it is within the grasp of all spiritual aspirants and yogis. It may be the most popular and respected philosophical work in India. The commentaries of Sankara, Ramanuja, and Madwacharya are very popular, as they interpret the Gita from the perspective of different schools of thought, such as Advaita (Monoism), Visishtadwaita (Qualified Monoism), and Dwaita (Dualism). Krishnamacharya gave considerable importance to the study of the Gita. Scores of contemporary writers have also written commentaries on this work, in several languages.

Siva Samhita—This is an important Siva yoga text; contains useful information on Hatha yoga. English translations are readily available.

Gheranda Samhita—Another Hatha yoga text, credited to a yogi called Gherunda Natha. Contains very useful information on Hatha yoga.

Isa Upanishad—One of the top ten Upanishads (Dasopanishad). Brief, but explains Brahman as the source of all.

Svetasvatara Upanishad—This is another Upanishad that is very well known, and is one of the Upanishads taught in detail to his students by Sri. T. Krishnamacharya. It has a good blend of Vedanta and yogic practices. The original text and English translations are readily available.

Chandogya Upanishad—One of the best known Upanishads from the Sama Veda. It contains several Upanishad Vidyas (discussions), such as Sad Vidya (knowledge of the essential), Dahara Vidya (knowledge of what resides in the heart's space), Bhuma Vidya (knowledge of the greatest), Panchagni Vidya (knowledge of the five transformations of the migrating soul). This Upanishad was one of Krishnamacharya's favorites. Many of the great saints, such as Sankara, have written detailed commentaries to this Upanishad.

Other Upanishads Sri. T. Krishnamacharya taught include Taittiriya, Brahad-Aranyaka, Prasna, Mandukya, Mundaka, and Sandlilya.

Yoga Taravali—A pithy work of Adi Sankara. It uses yoga methods to ultimately achieve moksha.

Thirumandiram—One of the most admired works by a Saivite saint called Tirumular, written in Tamil. It contains three thousand verses and one complete section on Ashtanga yoga. Some of the most complex ideas of the various Eastern philosophies, including yoga, are lucidly explained by the sage.

This is the goal of yoga according to the sage Patanjali, whose text Krishnamacharya took to be the ultimate authority on the subject. It differs from the goal of Hatha yoga, which is to unite the two energies symbolically represented by the sun (ha) and the moon (tha). Do these two goals amount to the same thing? A good question indeed.

Glossary of Sanskrit Terms/ English Index

Glossary/Index of Sanskrit Terms

This section is followed by the "English Index," an index of topics in English, starting on page 254.

239

243

245

Sanyasin—lit., one who has taken a vow to know and remain with the ultimate principle; the fourth stage of life; a renunciate, 45, 97, 155, 225, 230–31

Saphala—success, 169

Sarupya—lit., of the same form (of the Lord), 226

Sarvanga Sadhana—practice for all parts of the body, 150

Sarvangasana—all-body-parts pose/shoulder stand, 101–7, 206; benefits from, 146, 207; for chest colds, 209; for congestion in legs, 231; for insomnia, 207–8; as preparation for headstand, 82; timing in practice, 75–76; for uneven hips, 212; variations, 122; vinyasa method, 65–66, 77–78

Sastras—scriptures, 29, 53, 80; smritis, 25, 171, 173; swadhyaya, xxii, 4, 18–21, 22, 38, 220, 222. See also **Upanishad; Vedas**

Sat—truth, non-changing; existence, 14

Satchitananda—implies that Brahman is the source of existence, 14

Sathyakama—a sage, 171–72

Satva (or Sattwa)—one of the three gunas, the most beneficial to the individual in spiritual pursuit; it manifests as order, right conduct, piety, clarity of mind, lightness of body, and extraordinary achievements . . . distinction between purusha and chitta, 8, 12–13, 57; moving beyond the three gunas, 174, 219–20; as pure mind, 8, 17–18; and rajas, 73–74; rajas, tamas, and, 55, 157, 174–75; tamas as opposite, 77

Satwic—characteristic of light and clarity, 41–42, 227–28; practices for achieving, 124, 158, 160–61, 179; satwic food, 17–18; satwic mind, 10, 12–13, 18, 174–75; satwic people, 25, 34

Satwika Nidra—restful deep sleep, 182

Satya—truth, existence, eternity, 3, 31–33. See also **Yama Niyamas**

Saucha—cleanliness, 4. See also **Yama Niyamas**

Savasana—corpse pose, 87, 90, 197

Sayujya—merger with the Lord, 59, 226. See also **Moksha**

Shanmukha—six ports in the head/face, 198

Shanmukhi Mudra—sealing the six senses: the two eyes, the two ears, the nose and the mouth, 195–97; ending sessions with, 131, 208; for eye health, 121; as indicator of fitness, 101; for long periods of time, 146, 177; for short practices, 78, 231; uniting with agna chakra, 191; yoni mudra as same procedure, 198

Siddha—a person who has attained extraordinary achievements, 181–82

Siddhasana—a seated pose; a pose of accomplishment, 63, 152

Siddhi—accomplishment, 43, 105, 134, 140, 169, 181–82, 194; asana siddhi, 43–44

Simhasana—lion pose, 111, 208

Sirsasana—headstand, 88–89, 121–22, 156, 206; janu sirsana, 88, 117, 118

Sitali—breathing exercise that cools the system, 145

Siva Samhita—Hatha yoga text, 202

Siva—the destroyer, one of the trinity, 31–32, 89, 160, 164–65, 189

Smritis—texts written consistent with original scriptures, memories, 25, 171, 173

Sopasraya—with support, 116

Sthana—place, 66, 134, 203; kandasthana, 115, 146–47; lingasthana, 191; marmasthana, 198; pranasthana, 66; svadhishtana chakra, 187–92, 191

Sthira—steadiness, 122

Sthula Sarira—gross body, 53

Suddha—pure, 13

253

English Index